Vital Diabetes

GW00712282

Vital Diabetes

Your *essential* reference for
diabetes management in primary care

Second edition

Charles Fox BM, FRCP
Consultant Physician with Special Interest in Diabetes,
Northampton General Hospital Trust

and

Mary MacKinnon MMedSci, RGN
Senior Lecturer in Diabetes Care, and Director of Education,
Warwick Diabetes Care, University of Warwick

Class Health • London

Printing history
First published 1999
Reprinted 2000
Second edition 2002
Reprinted 2003

The authors and the publishers welcome feedback from the users of this book.
Please contact the publishers.
Class Publishing (London) Ltd, Barb House, Barb Mews, London W6 7PA
Telephone: 020 7371 2119; Fax: 020 7371 2878 [International +4420]
Email: post@class.co.uk; website: www.class.co.uk

A CIP catalogue record for this book is available from the British Library

ISBN 1 872362 93 1

Edited by Jane Sugarman

Designed and typeset by Martin Bristow

Printed and bound in Slovenia by Delo Tiskarna
by arrangement with Presernova druzba

Acknowledgements
We would like to thank Maria Mousley, specialist podiatrist in Northampton,
for her help with the foot-care section; Dr Ted Willis, GP, for his exacting
scrutiny of the page proofs; and our editor, Jane Sugarman.

Dear Colleagues

Welcome to *Vital Diabetes.*

This practical book is for you, working in general practice and in the community. Most of your local diabetes population has type 2 diabetes (formerly called non-insulin-dependent diabetes or NIDDM). *Vital Diabetes* concentrates on this serious medical condition, helping you to look after people with this type of diabetes and their near relatives, who also have an important role to play in health care. Treatment of type 1 diabetes (insulin-dependent diabetes – IDDM) is also mentioned.

The book gives you the vital information that you need in the practice or out in the community, tabbed for easy reference from the **section finder** (page 9). The detailed **contents list** (pages 6–8) allows you to pinpoint specific topics. The text is divided into ten distinct sections with topics clearly presented. At the end of each topic, we have put down one or more **vital points** that give you essential information in just a few words.

After most parts, you will find an associated page(s), called **patient and carer information**, which you can enlarge and photocopy for your patients. We would suggest that you enlarge this to A4 size.

You will find useful addresses and contact numbers at the end of the book, as well as references, further reading and details of training courses.

We hope that you will find this book helpful, time-saving and vital to your everyday clinical practice and that, in using it, you will be able to provide an up-to-date and consistent standard and quality of health care for people with diabetes.

Please use the form on page 95 for your feedback on *Vital Diabetes*. We would welcome your comments and suggestions for changes and improvements. Thank you.

Yours sincerely

Charles Fox and Mary MacKinnon

Contents

Section Finder

1 Impact and new insights

The impact of living with type 2 diabetes

'Diabetes is an easy disease to treat badly.'
Professor Robert Tattersall

The impact of a diagnosis of diabetes is very powerful and affects all aspects of a person's life, either in general (e.g. the possibility of reduced life expectancy) or in particular (e.g. the need to lose weight and keep to a healthy diet).

Most newly diagnosed patients with type 2 diabetes feel insecure. They are not sure about three important questions:

1. Whether or not they have a serious disorder.
2. Whether diabetes will interfere much with their lifestyle.
3. What they are expected to do about it.

Badly treated diabetes means patients are:

- Not being consulted about their ideas about diabetes.
- Ill-informed and unable to make choices about their own care.
- Not being involved or taking the lead in their own diabetes care plan.
- Not being the most valued and important member of their health care team.
- Being told that they have 'mild diabetes' which could have been avoided.
- Being unaware of the aim and possible consequences of their treatment.
- Made to feel censured if ideal weight is not achieved or maintained.
- Condemned for not achieving their target blood glucose level.
- Made to feel guilty – treatment failure is all their fault.
- Punished by the threat of insulin injections.
- Frightened at the prospect of insulin injections and the long-term complications of diabetes.

The result of badly treated diabetes is a life filled with fear and guilt. Personal relationships and relationships with health carers may be severely compromised and, occasionally, may break down completely.

Badly treated diabetes does not provide care for the person in the context of their cultural, psychological and social framework.

Well-treated diabetes involves patients:

- Being competently assessed on diagnosis by a properly trained person.
- Being aware of research activity and new insights in diabetes.
- Taking the lead and being involved in their own (staged) diabetes care plan, wherever possible.
- Being able to make informed choices about their own care.
- Feeling valued and that they are the most important member of the health care team.
- Knowing that type 2 diabetes is not 'mild' but a serious and complex medical condition with associated long-term complications.
- Knowing about long-term complications and how to reduce them.
- Understanding that type 2 diabetes cannot be cured but that it is not their fault.
- Knowing that the underlying causes are insulin resistance and progressive beta-cell (β-cell) failure – given explanation.
- Being informed that treatment may also be progressive and that insulin therapy may be required sooner rather than later, if optimum (agreed) blood glucose targets are not achieved.
- Knowing about the positive role of reduction in blood glucose and blood pressure levels in reducing the presence and severity of long-term complications.
- Feeling reassured, on diagnosis, that insulin injections are not to be feared – given a practical demonstration (even if diet-only treatment needed).
- Being aware of the risks and implications of medication and insulin therapy in the achievement of blood glucose and blood pressure (agreed) targets.
- Having their cultural differences recognised and incorporated into their diabetes care plans, as far as possible.
- Knowing that they are not alone; other people with diabetes can help.

- Knowing what care to expect, who will provide it and how, and where to get it locally.
- Understanding that most diabetes care is provided in the community and that secondary and tertiary services are involved, working with their general practice team.

Well treated, the impact of type 2 diabetes will also be reduced if relatives and carers are involved. They should aim to know as much as the person with diabetes and be consulted in order to provide the necessary standard of care for the person concerned.

Well-treated diabetes involves care for the person with sensitivity, embracing culture, psychological well-being, health beliefs and social structures in an individualised and thoughtful manner. The person with diabetes is central to care planning and is valued, well informed and able to make decisions on self-treatment and care.

VITAL POINTS: LIVING WITH TYPE 2 DIABETES

✶ Diabetes is a difficult disease, which can be well managed.
✶ Value the person with diabetes (and those close to them).
✶ Enable them to make their own decisions.

New insights into type 2 diabetes

There is continuing new evidence and insight into the management of type 2 diabetes. Four relevant studies have been completed and are summarised below.

1. United Kingdom Prospective Diabetes Study (UKPDS) (For references, see page 87)

Key points

- The largest clinical study of diabetes ever conducted.
- It studied the effect of intensive treatment of type 2 diabetes in reducing long-term complications.
- It demonstrated that long-term complications are reduced with intensive therapy.
- It found that a reduction in HbA1c of 1% was associated with 14% fewer myocardial infarctions, 21% fewer deaths related to diabetes and 37% fewer microvascular complications.
- It confirmed that type 2 diabetes is a serious and progressive disease and never 'mild'.
- It found that up to 50% of people with type 2 diabetes have long-term complications on diagnosis, emphasising the need for early detection and screening of those in high-risk groups.
- The key treatment targets, reducing long-term complications in the study, relate to tight blood pressure and intensive blood glucose control.

VITAL POINTS: UKPDS

* *Treatment targets (UKPDS) are:*
* *Blood pressure levels of < 130/80 mmHg.*
* *HbA1c levels of < 7.0%.*
* *Fasting blood glucose levels of 4–7 mmol/l.*
* *Self-monitored blood glucose levels before meals of between 4 and 7 mmol/l.*

2. Prevalence and incidence of type 2 diabetes in the UK (Poole 1998) (For references, see page 87)

- It is estimated that over 1 million people are currently diagnosed with type 2 diabetes in the UK.
- Another million may be undiagnosed.
- Over 100,000 people are diagnosed with diabetes each year in the UK (one person every five minutes).
- The number of cases among men is significantly higher than among women.
- This is a marked change from the position in the 1950s and 1960s, when cases among women were higher.
- The cause of this shift is unknown.
- Advancing age of the population, obesity and a sedentary lifestyle are thought to be contributing factors to increasing numbers of cases.
- Groups at particularly high risk are those aged over 40 years who are overweight or of Asian or Afro-Caribbean origin, or have a family history of diabetes or a prior history of gestational diabetes.

VITAL POINTS: INSIGHTS INTO TYPE 2 DIABETES

✻ Ensure that people are aware of diabetes symptoms, lifestyle factors and serious complications.

✻ Identify those at high risk.

✻ Provide best possible care to prevent the onset of complications.

3. Primary Care Diabetes – a national survey

(For references, see page 87)

A national survey in England and Wales (Pierce et al., 2000) aimed to describe the following:

- The extent and organisation of general practice diabetes care.
- Primary care perceptions of support by secondary care.
- Cooperation with secondary care.
- Educational experience in diabetes of doctors and nurses in primary care.

The enquiry confirmed that, over the past decade, the focus of diabetes care has shifted and most is provided in general practice. There are significant geographical variations in the delivery of primary diabetes care.

One in five practices in England and Wales was surveyed. The response to the survey was 70%.

Some results

- Median number of diabetes patients per practice is 110.
- 75% of patients with diabetes are described as having most or all of their diabetes care in general practice.
- 68% of practices had a special interest in diabetes.
- 96% of practices had diabetes registers.
- 87% of practices used their registers for call and recall.
- 77% of practices had fully computerised registers.

Key messages

- A large volume of diabetes care takes place in primary care.
- Those providing it are very enthusiastic.
- Nurses are important and the key to success.

VITAL POINTS: NATIONAL SURVEY FOR PCD

* Variations in primary diabetes care need exploring.
* Education for GPs and nurses needs development.

4. The Hypertension Optimal Treatment (HOT) Study

(For references, see page 87)

- A very large study (18,790 patients) to investigate the optimum target diastolic blood pressure.

- A subgroup of these hypertensive patients also had diabetes (1,501 patients).

- In patients with diabetes, a diastolic blood pressure of 80 mmHg led to a reduction of severe cardiovascular events by 51%, compared with a diastolic blood pressure of 90 mmHg.

- The reduction in morbidity was accompanied by a parallel improvement in well-being.

- UKPDS data (paper 36) show that patients with a normal systolic blood pressure (130 mmHg) have a lower risk of coronary heart disease.

- Thus, the target blood pressure for people with diabetes is 130/80.

2 Screening and identification

Screening

- The prevalence of diabetes in the UK is 3%.
- The prevalence increases with age: over 10% of people aged > 65 have diabetes.
- The prevalence in African, Asian and Afro-Caribbean people is > 6%.
- Up to 25% of people of Asian origin aged > 60 have diabetes.
- See the Diabetes UK Recommendations (2000) for the Management of Diabetes in Primary Care (resources list, page 87); these recommend that the people below should be screened for diabetes.

- All pregnant women.
- Patients with symptoms of:
    - thirst, polyuria and/or weight loss;
    - urinary symptoms, e.g. nocturia, urinary incontinence;
    - recurrent infections, especially of the skin;
    - pain, numbness and paraesthesiae (pins and needles);
    - visual changes;
    - mood changes;
    - tiredness, muscle weakness.
- People who are obese, especially central obesity (the apple-shaped body).
- People of Asian, African and Afro-Caribbean origin.
- People (all) aged over 65.
- Those with a family history of diabetes or cardiovascular disease.
- Women with a history of gestational diabetes or who have given birth to a large baby (birthweight > 4 kg).

- Screening should also be considered in patients with an underlying diagnosis of:
  - hypertension;
  - angina;
  - heart attack;
  - claudication;
  - stroke.

VITAL POINTS: SCREENING

People of Asian origin are more likely to develop type 2 diabetes and at an earlier age.

Flag the notes of those with a family history of diabetes.

Flag the notes of those with a history of gestational diabetes.

Screen those at risk of developing diabetes every 3 years.

Identification

- You should 'think diabetes'!
- Of a list of 2,000 patients, 60 are likely to have diabetes.
- About 80% of people with diabetes are managed in primary care, i.e. of 60 patients on your diabetes list, 48 will be managed in your practice.
- Of those presenting to your practice with diabetes, most will have type 2 diabetes (treated with diet, diet and tablets, or diet and insulin).
- Teach administrative staff (clerks/receptionists) about diabetes: to recognise the names of test strips, drugs and insulin on prescriptions, and identify people with diabetes on their notes.
- Give responsibility for people with diabetes to a 'named' person in the practice.
- Check that all staff have knowledge about diabetes.
- Check existing registers.
- Check prescription lists.
- Check existing 'labelled diabetes' patient records.
- Check patients new to the practice.

- Note those who are newly diagnosed.
- Be extra vigilant with those treated just by diet.
- Check records of regular home visits (for the housebound).
- Hang posters in the practice.
- Communicate with all members of the primary care team, especially those caring for people who are elderly or have mental illness/handicap.
- Contact the local pharmacist(s); they may know about the local diabetes population.

You need knowledge about:

- The total population covered by the practice.
- Percentage of elderly people (> 65 years) in the practice.
- Ethnic composition of the practice.

Finally:

- Add newly identified people with diabetes to your list.
- Label the patient records 'Diabetes'.
- Use this list as the basis of a diabetes register, whether on computer or paper.

Where and how people present in primary care

- At the surgery.
- In health promotion clinics.
- As new patients to the practice.
- At 'home' in screening programmes, e.g. for older people (> 75).
- At routine medical checks, e.g. for insurance purposes.
- To the community pharmacist, e.g. presenting with symptoms.
- After a visit to the optometrist (optician) and a routine vision check.
- At NHS walk-in centres.
- Via NHS Direct (telephone helpline).
- Self-diagnosis – anywhere.

Symptoms of type 2 diabetes: what to look for?

Symptoms (may develop slowly over months or years)

- Thirst
- Polyuria/nocturia
- Incontinence in elderly people
- Tiredness/lethargy
- Mood changes (irritability)
- Weight loss
- Visual disturbances
- Thrush infections (genital)
- Recurrent infections (boils/ulcers)
- Tingling/pain/numbness (in feet, legs, hands)
- Unexplained symptoms

DIABETES – DO YOU SUFFER FROM

- **Excessive thirst?**
- **Going to the toilet to pass water (a lot)?**
- **Blurred vision?**
- **Itching 'down below'?**
- **Tiredness?**
- **Weight loss?**
- **Mood changes?**
- **Weight gain?**

**IF YOU DO,
PLEASE LET US KNOW**

You might want to produce a poster like this to encourage people with undiagnosed diabetes to come forward. Alternatively, you can obtain such a poster from Diabetes UK (see page 90).

Diagnostic criteria

- Diagnosis of diabetes has important legal and medical implications so diagnosis must be definite.
- Do not base diagnosis on glycosuria or stick reading of finger-prick blood glucose; use only for screening.
- Measurement of HbAlc is not currently recommended for screening.
- Diabetes should be confirmed on a venous plasma blood sample sent to a laboratory.
- Diabetes is confirmed by:
  - random plasma blood glucose concentration of ≥ 11.1 mmol/l or
  - fasting plasma glucose concentration of ≥ 7.0 mmol/l or
  - 2-hour plasma glucose concentration of ≥ 11.1 mmol/l, 2 hours after 75 g glucose in an oral glucose tolerance test (OGTT).
- Some people with glycosuria have impaired glucose tolerance diagnosed by an OGTT, organised with the local laboratory.
- HbA1c should be measured as a baseline recording.
- Refer children with suspected diabetes urgently: don't wait for results of diagnostic tests.

VITAL POINTS: DIAGNOSTIC CRITERIA

✱ Any child in whom a diagnosis of diabetes is suspected should be referred urgently by telephone to a hospital paediatric department for confirmation of diagnosis.

✱ Pay attention to cardiovascular risk factors, and survey annually for development of diabetes.

Impaired fasting glucose and impaired glucose tolerance

- Close monitoring of people with impaired glucose homeostasis is recommended (by the WHO Expert Committee).
- There are two categories of glucose homeostasis: impaired glucose tolerance (IGT) and a new category of impaired fasting glycaemia (IFG).
- IGT is defined by a 2-hour glucose during an oral glucose tolerance test (OGTT) of $\geq$ 7.8 mmol/l, but < 11.1 mmol/l, or a fasting plasma glucose of < 7.0 mmol/l.
- IFG is defined by a fasting glucose of $\geq$ 6.1 to < 7 mmol/l.
- Two abnormal test results on two different days are needed to confirm the diagnosis.
- Those diagnosed as having IGT and IFG are at risk of developing diabetes later in life; they should be advised about lifestyle and dietary points to lessen the risk.
- Such people need to be screened for diabetes every 3 years.
- Screen the same people for cardiovascular disease.

VITAL POINT: IFG AND IGT

* *Many people with IGT (and gestational diabetes) are likely to develop type 2 diabetes in later life and deserve regular screening.*

Criteria for referral

Criteria for referral to a diabetes specialist team need to be locally agreed between primary and secondary care providers.

- If someone with diabetes is ill and the diabetes cannot be controlled.
- If insulin treatment is needed (with urgent referral in the newly diagnosed person) and locally agreed. For type 1 this should be within 24 hours.
- If the condition of the feet of the person with diabetes is deteriorating.
- If there are any of the following complications:
  - uncontrolled hypertension;
  - sexual dysfunction;
  - persistent proteinuria;
  - rising creatinine levels;
  - unexplained loss of vision;
  - deteriorating retinopathy;
  - painful neuropathy, mononeuropathy, amyotrophy.
- If there are psychological problems, such as:
  - failure to accept diagnosis;
  - morbid fear of complications;
  - family difficulties.
- If a pregnancy is planned.
- Immediate hospital referral (see page 76) is needed for:
  - protracted vomiting – an emergency referral is required;
  - moderate or heavy ketonuria/evidence of ketoacidosis;
  - an acutely infected or ischaemic foot;
  - the newly diagnosed (type 1);
  - an unplanned pregnancy.

VITAL POINT: REFERRAL CRITERIA

* *Criteria for referral need to be explicitly locally agreed between primary and secondary care.*

Myths and misconceptions

It is important to recognise that, in all long-term disease, myths and misconceptions, preconceived ideas, education and life experience form the basis of individual health beliefs. This is particularly true at the time of diagnosis, when attitudes to the concept of a life-long incurable medical condition are set into place.

In diabetes, myths and misconceptions abound.

Myths and misconceptions

✱ Diabetes can be cured.
✱ Type 2 diabetes is a 'mild' condition.
✱ It is caused by eating too much sugar.
✱ It is the patient's fault.
✱ Dietary treatment means severe restriction.
✱ Specialist diabetic foods will be essential.
✱ If insulin is required, the diabetes is more severe.

Breaking the news

- Once people have been diagnosed with diabetes, sit them down, and give them time to digest the information.
- Explain that diabetes is a life-long condition and ask them how they feel about this.
- Ask them what they know about diabetes.
- Discuss their fears and myths/misconceptions about the condition (in an informal way).
- Ask them if they are aware of any family history, e.g. Auntie X had her leg amputated.
- The family or carer needs to be involved in the discussions, so, if not present, suggest that an early appointment is made for the family to come along as well; after all, others may very well be involved with cooking meals.
- Give small amounts of information and frequent appointments, so that they can absorb the information more easily.
- Arrange the next appointment straight away.
- Remember that the person's perception about diabetes affects how they cope in this initial period immediately after diagnosis.
- Explain the symptoms of diabetes and assure them that they can be quickly relieved; diabetes is a controllable long-term condition.
- Give people with diabetes and their families non-judgemental support that is positive and on-going.
- Give them a simple explanation of the physiology of diabetes and its treatment at an early appointment.
- Reinforce the person's desire to take care of him- or herself.

VITAL POINTS: BREAKING THE NEWS

* *Don't bombard a patient with information.*
* *Give plenty of time for him or her to deal with it.*

The next page can be copied and given to the patient so that he or she knows what to expect and what is expected of him or her.

Patient and carer information: what is diabetes?

- In type 2 diabetes the amount of sugar (glucose) in your blood is too high because the body is unable to use it properly.
- Insulin is the hormone that helps the sugar called glucose to get into the cells where it is used for energy.
- Insulin also stops the over-production of glucose by the liver.
- The main symptoms are increased thirst, passing large quantities of urine, extreme tiredness, weight loss, general itching and blurred vision.
- Type 2 diabetes develops when either your body does not produce enough insulin, or insulin produced does not work properly – insulin resistance.
- The main aims of treatment are:
  - achieving near normal blood sugar (glucose) levels and living a healthy lifestyle which will help you to feel better;
  - improving your blood pressure by ensuring that it is checked and that you are taking any prescribed tablets;
  - protecting you against long-term damage to the eyes, kidneys, nerves, heart and major arteries (blood vessels).
- When you have been diagnosed, you should have:
  - a full medical examination;
  - a talk with a registered nurse with a special interest in diabetes;
  - a talk with a state-registered dietitian;
  - a discussion about the implications of your diabetes for your job, driving, insurance and prescription charges;
  - information about Diabetes UK, their services and your local group;
  - continuing education about your diabetes.
- Dependent on your treatment you should also have the following:
  - if you are treated with diet alone, instructions on blood or urine tests and how to interpret the results, and supplies of equipment;
  - if you are treated with tablets, the above plus additional discussions about hypoglycaemia ('hypos' = low blood sugar) and how to deal with them;
  - if you are treated with insulin, both of the above plus a session on injection technique, looking after insulin and syringes, and also blood sugar (glucose) testing;
  - information about what can happen to your diabetes control during illness.

3 How to manage type 2 diabetes

The metabolic syndrome

Also known as syndrome X and Reaven's syndrome, the metabolic syndrome is a complex condition that is associated with:

- insulin resistance and type 2 diabetes;
- hypertension;
- central obesity;
- hyperlipidaemia;
- hyperinsulinaemia;
- polycystic ovary syndrome.

At the heart of this syndrome is the problem of insulin resistance. This is a vicious circle. Insulin resistance can lead to weight gain, which in turn worsens insulin resistance.

Insulin resistance

- Insulin resistance is one of the fundamental defects of type 2 diabetes.
- Insulin resistance is an early feature of the development of type 2 diabetes.
- The body fails to respond to its own insulin. This can initially be compensated for by an increase in insulin secretion.
- Insulin-resistant patients may become hyperinsulinaemic.
- Continued insulin resistance leads to the eventual exhaustion of the pancreatic beta cells. This results in a failure to produce adequate insulin and a further increase in blood glucose.
- In type 2 diabetes, insulin resistance is characterised by: impaired (insulin-stimulated) glucose uptake by fat, liver and skeletal muscle, and over-production of glucose by the liver.
- Insulin resistance is central to the development of cardiovascular risk factors, which are clustered together in the metabolic syndrome described earlier.

- Regular vigorous exercise improves oxygen consumption and reduces insulin resistance, even in elderly people.
- The problems caused by insulin resistance can be reduced by lifestyle changes.
- Thiazolidinediones (also called PPAR-gamma agonists or glitazones) are new drugs that target insulin resistance. They improve glycaemic control by improving insulin sensitivity at key sites of insulin resistance - namely fat, liver and skeletal muscle.

VITAL POINT: INSULIN RESISTANCE

* Insulin resistance is one of the fundamental defects of type 2 diabetes.

Hypertension: treatment plans

- Raised blood pressure is very common in type 2 diabetes (40-50%).
- There is increasing evidence that aggressive BP treatment reduces vascular complications in diabetes.
- As a result, the threshold for starting treatment and the target for treatment are both falling.
- Start treatment if systolic BP > 150 or diastolic BP > 90 mmHg.
- Aim at normalising blood pressure (130/80), using HOT Study targets (see page 16).
- Treat older people with equal enthusiasm, because they are more likely to derive early benefits.

Drugs used to treat hypertension

- There is evidence that ACE (angiotensin-converting enzyme) inhibitors have a protective effect on kidneys in people with diabetes, and possibly reduce retinopathy over and above their effect in reducing blood pressure.
- The UKPDS (UK Prospective Diabetes Study) found that ACE inhibitors confer no greater benefit than beta blockers in hypertension. However, the UKPDS carries the simple messages:

- high BP is common in type 2 diabetes;
- tight BP control has a major effect in reducing complications, including retinopathy;
- many patients need two or more drugs to achieve the target BP of 130/80.

- Doctors should continue using the antihypertensive drugs that they are familiar with, remembering that (in hypertension) compliance may be improved if a drug needs to be taken only once daily.

- All drugs used for treating hypertension have well-recognised side effects:
  - thiazides: low serum K^+, raised blood glucose and impotence;
  - beta blockers: may worsen asthma and peripheral vascular disease;
  - ACE inhibitors: cough; in rare cases, they can cause renal failure; angioneurotic oedema;
  - calcium blockers: flushing, headache, oedema.

Risk factors for coronary heart disease

Increased concentrations of LDL cholesterol

Decreased concentrations of HDL cholesterol

Hyperglycaemia (HbA1c > 6.2%)

Insulin resistance

Hypertension

Smoking

Being male

VITAL POINTS: HYPERTENSION

* Educate patients about the importance of BP in diabetes.

* Check BP at every clinic visit in all patients – especially if there is proteinuria.

* Aim for a target BP of 130/80.

Assessing and examining the newly diagnosed patient

Assessment, examination and tests for newly diagnosed person with diabetes should be sensitive to the individual and carried out in stages.

- Discuss general aspects of diabetes, enquire about any family history and history of illness leading to diagnosis.
- Listen and respond to preconceived ideas and anxieties. Establish existing knowledge of diabetes.
- Give simple explanation of diabetes, and discuss any fears that the patient may have and answer questions.
- Discuss general health and make next appointment.

- Weigh patient and measure height. Calculate body mass index (BMI) and agree target for ideal body weight.
  BMI = Weight in kilograms/(Height in metres)^2, that is, kg/m^2.
- Measure blood pressure.
- Examine for complications of diabetes: lower limbs; peripheral pulses and sensation; visual acuity; fundoscopy with dilated pupils. Unless you are entirely confident about fundoscopy, enrol patient in retinal screening programme.
- Test urine for glucose, ketones and protein.
- Test blood for fasting glucose, renal function, HbA1c.
- Measure fasting cholesterol and triglyceride levels; this should be done after a period of treatment because initial high triglycerides may improve with better blood glucose control.
- Consider arranging the following tests and reconsider at each annual review: full blood count; ECG; liver function tests; blood; thyroid function tests. Make next appointment.

- Discuss all results from previous visit and lifestyle in relation to diabetes; record drinking and smoking, advise strongly against the latter.

- Discuss food and meal planning, and initiate advice regarding eating plan.
- Arrange prescription (if required) and next appointment – regular and early reviews will be necessary until the patient has a good understanding of diabetes and metabolic control is achieved.
- Record information in the practice records and in diabetes cooperation cards, if used.
- Enter patient details on practice diabetes register.
- Notify information to district diabetes register.
- Patients must be informed if data held on a register outside the practice.

Assessment checklist at diagnosis and annual review

- Demographic information/changes
- Family status/changes
- Employment status/changes
- Medical history/changes
- Lifestyle history/changes
- Diabetes management/changes.

VITAL POINTS: ASSESSMENT

* Spending time with the patient is an investment in preventing complications and maintaining well-being in the future.

* A trusting, therapeutic relationship is vital to encourage continuity of health care.

What to do next: ongoing management plan

For the primary care team this follows:

- Full medical examination on diagnosis.
- All patients with diabetes need an annual review, including the measurement of HbA1c and screening for complications.
- Review all patients with diabetes 3- to 6-monthly to assess control of blood glucose, blood pressure and side effects of treatment.
- Management aims:
  - relief of symptoms;
  - discussion of potential side effects of treatment, especially hypos;
  - reduction in risks of acute complications;
  - identification of long-term complications as early as possible;
  - ensure that the patient has a satisfactory lifestyle.
- Support, advise and educate the person with diabetes about treatment.
- Negotiate appropriate targets for control and treatment.
- Assess regularly the symptoms and well-being of person with diabetes.
- Provide initial and continuing education to people with diabetes and their carers.
- Provide information about social and economic support.

The next page can be copied and given to the patient so that he or she knows what to expect and what is expected of him or her.

Patient and carer information: first steps

- Find out all you can about diabetes and check with your care team.
- Inform others about your diabetes: your family, friends and work colleagues.
- Attend for regular checks.
- Be in control of your diabetes on a daily basis.
- Monitor your own sugar levels and change treatment as advised.
- Keep a record of your blood (or urine) tests.
- Know when to seek help and where, particularly in an emergency or if you are ill.
- Discuss your fears with your team.
- Ask questions and repeat if not answered; prepare them before your appointment.
- Follow a healthy lifestyle: choosing healthy food, controlling your weight, taking physical exercise and not smoking.
- Examine your feet regularly. If you find this difficult, try to arrange for someone to do this.
- Recognise signs of low/high blood glucose levels and how to prevent.
- Be aware of the long-term complications of diabetes, the importance of early detection and the relevance of reducing blood glucose (sugar) levels to reduce the risk of complications.
- Inform the DVLA (tel: 01792 772151) and your insurance company if you drive.
- Carry personal identification (Medic-Alert) and warning card with details of who can help.
- If you are female and hoping to have a baby, get advice on your diabetes before trying to conceive.
- Consider joining Diabetes UK to keep you updated re diabetes.

Routine review

- Ensure that patients with established diabetes are included on the diabetes register and are booked for regular appointments.
- Organise a system for identifying and recalling defaulters and agree a policy for the frequency of follow-up of people with diabetes.
- Routine visits may be required two or three times a year in patients whose management and understanding of the condition are established.
- Make time to discuss the patient's attitude to diabetes and general well-being, enquire about any problems (life changes, hypos, diet, etc.). If treated with insulin, check injection sites.
- Most patients will have times in their lives when their diabetes is difficult to control, i.e. family crisis, other health problems, etc.
- Identify those who may be having problems on a regular basis and discuss with the patient how to deal with this.
- Weigh patient.
- Measure blood pressure and start treatment if raised.
- Test urine for glucose, ketones and protein; check mid-stream urine (MSU) if protein present.
- Take a blood sample for HbA1c (it makes sense to take this, and any other blood samples, 7 days before review appointment so that results are available for discussion with patient).
- Identify and discuss any weak spots in knowledge of diabetes and self-management skills.
- Make it clear that the patient should return if there are problems with hypos, high sugar levels or side effects – set agreed limits.
- Discuss and agree targets with the patient relating to their records of blood or urine tests, altering therapy as required.
- Record all details in diabetes record card and/or practice record.
- Arrange next appointment.

VITAL POINT: ROUTINE REVIEW

* *Patients who take part in regular structured care have better metabolic control and less risk of complications.*

Annual review

- Enquire about life events:
  - subjective changes in eyes and feet;
  - claudication;
  - neuropathic symptoms, impotence;
  - chest pain, shortness of breath.
- Discuss the patient's general progress and well-being, enquire about any problems relating to diabetes, in particular hypos or side effects of drugs. If treated with insulin, check injection sites.
- Weigh patient.
- Urinalysis: glucose/albumin/ketones. In type 2 patients with no ischaemic heart disease need to check that no microalbuminuria (risk factor).
- Arrange MSU if protein/blood present.
- Examine for diabetic complications:
  - blood pressure;
  - visual acuity;
  - eyes: refer for screening;
  - arrange MSU, if appropriate;
  - feet: general condition, pulses, ulceration; sensation.
- Review and agree targets with patient relating to their blood (or urine) tests.
- Take blood sample for:
  - blood glucose (feed back result);
  - HbA1c (performed in advance of annual review);
  - creatinine (if proteinuria is present);
  - cholesterol (every three years if normal);

  these tests should be performed in advance of the annual review.
- Check and discuss management with patient: dietary; treatment; targets; risk factors for heart disease and other long-term complications; management plan, including contraception and plans for pregnancies in women – altering therapy as required.
- Record information in the records, practice diabetes register and patient cooperation card if used.
- Arrange prescription (if required) and next appointment.
- Notify information to the district diabetes register.

Patient and carer information: ongoing management

Once your diabetes is controlled:

- You should be able to see the diabetes team regularly and be able to discuss problems and diabetes control.
- You should also be able to get in touch with any member of the team for specialist advice.
- You will have more education sessions.
- You will attend a medical review with a doctor or trained nurse once a year; this will involve the following:
  - being weighed;
  - a test of your urine for protein;
  - a test of your blood to check long-term glucose control;
  - a measurement of blood pressure;
  - a discussion about glucose control;
  - a check of your vision and examination of the back of your eyes, with a photo possibly being taken; if any significant problems are found you will be referred to an ophthalmologist;
  - an examination of your legs and feet;
  - an opportunity to discuss how you are coping at home and work.

Education checklist: the primary care team

Checklist of items to be discussed with patients:

- What is diabetes?
- Diet
- Tablets
- Insulin and injection technique
- Hypoglycaemia
- Hyperglycaemia
- Illness
- Blood testing
- Urine testing
- Foot care
- Importance of eye checks
- Smoking
- Alcohol
- Exercise
- Complications
- Driving/insurance
- Sexual health
- Planning pregnancy
- Diabetes UK
- Free prescriptions
- Benefits.

Although most patients can usually control their blood glucose by diet and/or tablets at the onset, this becomes more difficult with time. This is a result of beta-cell failure and progressive insulin resistance and is not the patient's fault. Many people with type 2 diabetes end up needing insulin; the average time from diagnosis is 7 years.

VITAL POINT: IMPORTANT PRIMARY CARE POINT

* *Type 2 diabetes is a progressive condition.*

Patient and carer information: lifestyle issues

General advice

- You have a vital part to play in your own treatment and management.
- Eat regular meals.
- Avoid being overweight.
- Eat more high-fibre and starchy foods, such as wholemeal bread, cereals.
- Eat less sugary foods, such as sweetened drinks, cakes, chocolate.
- Cut down on the amount of fat that you eat.
- Go easy on the amount of salt you use.
- Drink alcohol in moderation.
- Avoid special diabetic products: they can be high in fat and cost more.
- DO NOT SMOKE.
- Take regular exercise.
- If you follow the above, by eating healthily and exercising you will be able to lower your blood sugar (glucose) levels.
- By keeping your blood glucose levels in the normal range you can have a long and healthy life.
- If you still have levels of blood glucose that are too high, you may need to take insulin as well as the tablets.
- Check your feet and footwear regularly; keep your feet clean.
- Get your eyes checked regularly: you are entitled to a free eye check every year if you take tablets or insulin for your diabetes.
- Know what to do if you are ill or have a 'hypo'.
- You do not have to pay for prescriptions if you are on tablets or insulin.

Meal planning advice

This list gives advice about the way in which your meals should be planned.

- Maintain a constant intake of energy (i.e. eat regularly) as fluctuations have an effect on blood glucose levels.
- Eat regular meals.
- Don't eat a lot of foods that are high in energy, such as fatty meat, fried foods, dairy products and sugary foods and drinks as they result in poor blood sugar (glucose) control.
- Half your energy intake should come from starches such as bread, potatoes, rice, pasta, cereals, beans and lentils.
- Eat high-fibre foods (such as whole-grain bread, jacket potatoes).
- Beans, lentils, oats and citrus fruits have been shown to promote a slow, steadier rise in blood sugar levels.
- Keep carbohydrates such as sweets, chocolates and sweet drinks for special occasions, emergencies such as hypoglycaemia ('hypo') or illness, or as a snack before strenuous activity.
- Ask for advice if you need to lose weight.
- Work with a dietitian or practice nurse to plan your meals.
- Eat less fat.
- Eat less salt.
- Control your alcohol intake: a maximum of three 'units' for men and two for women per day is recommended (1 'unit' = half pint of ordinary beer or lager or small glass of wine or a single measure of spirits).
- Don't buy special diabetic foods: they are expensive and often high in fat; they may contain sorbitol, which can cause diarrhoea.

Weight control advice

- The more weight you carry, the greater the problem with insulin resistance, which leads to increased glucose levels. Even a small weight reduction can improve this.
- By controlling your weight you may put off the need for tablets, as diabetes can be controlled by diet for longer.
- You can control your weight through diet and through exercise or activity.
- Itemise your diet and discuss with the appropriate experts how you can adjust it to help you meet your goals/targets.
- Ask for help and encouragement from family and friends.
- Find a realistic routine that suits you.
- Enjoy what you do eat, and make allowances for occasional lapses.
- If you aim to lose weight, you may need to reduce your tablets/insulin. Discuss this with your diabetes care team.

Exercise/activity advice

- The Health Education Authority recommends that you have 30 minutes of moderate physical exercise/activity on at least 5 days a week.
- This will improve your health.
- Build up to this target gradually, not in 1 or 2 weeks.
- Consider ways in which you can make exercise part of your daily routine.
- Moderate activity is activity that raises your heartbeat and makes you feel warm and slightly out of breath (with the emphasis on slightly).
- Physical activity includes gardening, brisk walking, cycling, swimming, dancing and various sports.
- Do not take up strenuous activity unless you have been examined by a doctor and pronounced fit.
- By exercising and improving your health, you can:
  - manage the stresses of life;
  - control your blood pressure;
  - reduce your risk of heart disease;
  - prevent brittle bones in later life;
  - reduce the risks of some cancers;
  - keep mobile and independent in later life.

Alcohol advice

Alcohol stops the production of glucose by the liver for up to 12 hours, even though the level of sugar in the bloodstream may rise immediately after drinking alcohols with high carbohydrate levels.

- All the rules about alcohol that apply to everyone apply to you.

- Too much alcohol (whether high carbohydrate ones such as beer and lager or those containing no carbohydrates such as spirits or low-calorie mixers) may cause a hypo, particularly if you take insulin.

- Some alcohol contains a lot of calories so heavy drinking will make you overweight, leading to poor sugar (glucose) control and poor health. But you can still have a hypo.

- If and when you drink, avoid low-sugar beers which are higher in alcohol content and low-alcohol beers which are high in sugar; go for ordinary beers, and avoid drinks that are high in sugar (sweet wine/sherry/liqueurs).

- Use mixers or soft drinks that are diet, low calorie or sugar free.

- Know your drinks and check the percentage alcohol content.

- Limit your drinking to two (women) or three (men) units a day (1 unit = half a pint of beer, a glass of wine or a pub measure of spirits).

- If you take insulin, don't drink on an empty stomach.

- Eat little and often while you are drinking.

- Always carry glucose tablets or sweets.

- Always wear or carry your diabetes information as a hypo can be confused with drunkenness.

- Hypos can happen the morning after an evening drinking session.

- Avoid alcohol if you are pregnant as it could harm your baby.

Cultural issues

- Be aware of different cultures and religions and how they can affect many aspects, from the way in which you talk to a patient on initial presentation, to the advice that you give about diet and lifestyle issues.

- Be aware of the differences in etiquette that are necessary in examination of patients from different cultures.

- Have respect for the individual's culture/lifestyle.

- Find out about the customs for communicating with patients from ethnic minorities and about their customs and dietary rules.

- There are many cultural differences with regard to food and these need to be remembered when the person with diabetes is from a different culture.

- Be aware that in some communities it is believed that certain foods are 'hot' whereas others are 'cold' – during certain illnesses, only one type will be eaten.

- Remember that people from ethnic minorities have particular dietary habits and eat foods that are of cultural importance, e.g. ghee and sweetmeats among Asian communities (Hindu and Moslem), halal meat (Moslem), kosher food (Jewish), etc. These need to be considered when advice is given about diet.

- Be aware of the traditional/herbal medicines that are used within some Afro-Asian communities as some of them can cause hypoglycaemia or may be toxic to the liver. Ask patients about their use.

- The practice should organise a link worker for different ethnic groups.

- In some cultures, the idea of self-injection is anathema. Take this into consideration and suggest a third party to take responsibility for insulin injections.

Treatment

Aims

- Relief of symptoms.
- A satisfactory lifestyle.
- Prevention of unwanted effects of treatment (i.e. hypoglycaemia, side effects of drugs).
- Reduction of the risks of acute complications (hypoglycaemia, hyperglycaemia).
- Reduction of the risks of long-term complications, such as coronary heart disease, visual impairment, amputation and renal failure.

Targets for good blood glucose control

- The targets for good diabetic control are fasting blood glucose (FBG, finger prick test) < 6 mmol/l and HbA1c < 7%. The UKPDS has demonstrated two important points:
  - patients who achieve these targets have a lower risk of developing complications
  - type 2 diabetes is a progressive disorder caused by insulin resistance and increasing loss of insulin production by the pancreas.
- Total blood glucose load over time is a major risk factor for vascular disease and diabetic complications.
- At the onset, patients find it easy to control blood glucose within tight limits.
- UKPDS has shown that most patients progress from a single tablet regimen, through to combination regimens and potentially to insulin therapy to ensure tight glycaemic control.
- The average time from diagnosis to needing insulin is 7 years. Goals are set for patients, which are increasingly hard to achieve because of risk or fear of hypos or unacceptable weight gain.
- Patients need to be told this sobering information and reassured that, when and if they come to need insulin, it is because their diabetes is getting worse and not through any fault of their own.

Treatment plan for type 2 diabetes

- Given the progressive nature of type 2 diabetes, patients tend to feel that they have let us or themselves down when they are unable to maintain tight blood glucose control.

- In the treatment cascade below, patients have to buy into each step. There is no point in 'bouncing' a reluctant patient on to insulin treatment, and a few months of poor control will not be harmful. The whole process may take many years and each step should be taken slowly and carefully with patient and carers being fully informed.

- If the targets are achieved, review in 3–6 months.

VITAL POINTS: INITIAL TREATMENT

✻ Diet is the first line of treatment for type 2 diabetes.
✻ If possible avoid tablets for the first 3 months.

The treatment cascade

✻ Diet for a period of 3 months. Lose weight if overweight.
✻ Add metformin or a sulphonylurea if diet or exercise fail.
✻ Increase dose of tablets as necessary.
✻ Add another oral medication.
✻ Combination insulin and oral medication.
✻ Insulin therapy alone.

Treatment with tablets

Metformin

- First-line treatment especially in **overweight patients** with type 2 diabetes.

- Main action is to decrease hepatic glucose output.

- Side effects are common and occur in 30% of patients prescribed metformin, and include nausea, flatulence, diarrhoea, constipation, anorexia, metallic taste and impaired absorption of vitamin B_{12}.

- Take with food to minimise side effects.

- Start with one tablet a day and build up the dose gradually.
- Lactic acidosis is a rare but serious complication.
- Avoid in cardiac failure or renal impairment.
- Not safe if liver tests are abnormal, e.g. in alcoholism.
- Avoid in women who are pregnant or breast-feeding.

VITAL POINT: TREATMENT WITH METFORMIN

* *Avoid metformin in people with failure of the heart, kidneys or liver.*

Sulphonylureas

- Often used in **normal weight patients** with type 2 diabetes, although metformin can be equally effective in normal weight patients.
- Stimulate insulin release from the pancreas.
- Potent drugs, which may cause profound hypoglycaemia, particularly when first introduced.
- If hypoglycaemia occurs, reduce dose.
- May induce weight gain, as a result of the anabolic effect of insulin.
- Avoid in women who are pregnant or breast-feeding.
- Use with caution in elderly people with diabetes and those with renal failure.
- Side effects are mild and infrequent: rashes, headache and, very rarely, blood disorders.
- Glibenclamide is now less widely used because of the risk of dangerous long-lasting hypos.
- Gliclazide is safer in renal failure and appears to cause fewer hypos in elderly people with diabetes.
- Glimepiride is a new generation, long-acting, single-dose sulphonylurea. It has the advantage of being taken as a single dose.

VITAL POINTS: TREATMENT WITH SULPHONYLUREAS

* *Avoid all tablets in pregnant women.*
* *All sulphonylureas can cause hypos.*

Thiazolidinediones

- Add-on treatments. Approved by NICE (National Institute for Clinical Excellence) in combination therapy but not as a first-line treatment and not in combination with insulin therapy.
- Act by improving insulin resistance, the root cause of type 2 diabetes.
- Reduce blood glucose and insulin levels by increasing effectiveness of available insulin in liver, fat and muscle.
- Potentiate the action of both the body's own insulin and also injected insulin.
- Rosiglitazone (GlaxoSmithKline) was launched in the UK in July 2000. Published data and clinical trials have indicated no adverse effects on the liver to date. It is recommended, however, that LFTs (Liver Function Tests) are performed prior to the commencement of therapy, two monthly for the first year, and periodically thereafter. It can be used in combination with metformin or sulphonylureas in certain circumstances, but is not yet licensed for use in combination with insulin.
- Pioglitazone (Takeda) was launched in November 2000. Use is as for rosiglitazone.
- Thiazolidinediones are well tolerated and, because of their mechanism of action, cannot cause hypos when given alone (i.e. as a first-line treatment).
- Side effects are minimal. They may include weight gain and ankle swelling (dilutional anaemia) unrelated to heart failure

Postprandial glucose regulators

- Postprandial glucose regulators (PPGRs, e.g. repaglinide) are taken immediately before a meal.
- If a meal is missed, then it is not necessary to take a dose.
- PPGRs work like a sulphonylurea, with a faster onset and shorter duration of action.
- They can be introduced when diet and exercise are no longer adequate.
- They can be used when metformin monotherapy is insufficient.
- Incidence of hypos is less with PPGRs than with sulphonylureas.

Combination of drugs

- As type 2 diabetes is a progressive disease, combination therapy is increasingly seen as the preferred method of treatment to maintain good glycaemic control.
- A combination of metformin and a thiazolidinedione or a sulphonylurea and a thiazolidinedione is approved by NICE.
- Metformin causes gastrointestinal side effects and people often feel better after starting insulin.
- The UKPDS demonstrated the importance of tight blood glucose control in reducing or delaying long-term complications of type 2 diabetes. Thus patients with HbA1c > 7.5% on a combination of tablets should consider the need for insulin.
- People with diabetes often have other risk factors, such as hypertension or raised lipids, and need to take additional medication to reduce these risks.
- Tablet boxes to organise daily medication are available from chemists.

VITAL POINTS: COMBINATION TREATMENT (DRUGS)

* *The UKPDS showed that tight blood glucose control is important in reducing or delaying long-term complications of type 2 diabetes.*

* *It does not matter how this is achieved.*

* *Any reduction in glycated haemoglobin (HbA1c) will be beneficial in the reduction of long-term complications.*

* *Don't be afraid to try any combination of therapies to achieve the desired result.*

Combination with insulin

- Traditionally, people with type 2 diabetes have been treated with tablets for as long as possible and then changed over to insulin.
- A new and acceptable approach is combination therapy with tablets and insulin.
- This helps people become accustomed to insulin injections and to adjusting the dose according to their blood glucose tests.
- Start by adding a long-acting insulin at bedtime (say 10 units) and monitoring the early morning glucose.
- The final dose of insulin needed to achieve a morning glucose < 6 mmol/l will depend mainly on body weight.
- The dose of insulin should be increased steadily until the target is achieved.
- Metformin or sulphonylureas should be continued at the previous dose, which should be more effective if the fasting glucose is well controlled.
- As the beta cells in the pancreas cease to function, daytime blood glucose levels will creep up, resulting in a rise in HbA1c.
- At some stage, tablets have little useful effect and the person will have to move over to two or more daily injections of insulin.

Note that, at each stage in this process, the person with diabetes and the clinic team must decide whether or not to move on to the next stage. Many people, particularly if elderly or very overweight, may be better off accepting less than ideal metabolic control. In the UKPDS, the benefits of tight control were not seen for about 6 years. So, in people with a life expectancy shorter than this, there is no point in struggling for perfection.

VITAL POINT: COMBINATION TREATMENT (INSULIN)

✳ Combination therapy with a bedtime dose of insulin suits many people – it provides a gentle introduction to full-blown insulin therapy.

Insulin in type 2 diabetes

- Insulin therapy should be considered in type 2 diabetes when:
  - symptoms persist;
  - blood glucose levels are high – HbA1c > 7.5%;
  - there is an intercurrent illness or a need for steroid therapy.
- Decision to move over to insulin therapy:
  - when there are symptoms of thirst, tiredness, itchy genitalia;
  - depends on body weight: it is difficult to treat very obese patients with insulin.
- Success factors for insulin therapy:
  - when a person is committed to good control;
  - depends on family history: parents or siblings are on insulin;
  - when workmates or friends are on insulin – they may encourage someone to 'take the plunge'.
- HbA1c is the best indicator of metabolic control. Inform patients of the local threshold and about progressive loss of insulin production by the pancreas.
- Treatment with insulin should start with a small dose of insulin – usually 10 units twice daily of long-acting or pre-mixed insulin.
- Overweight patients will need larger doses.
- Those who measure their own blood glucose can be taught to increase their dose in response to the level. They may want to discuss changes with their care team.
- Most people with type 2 diabetes achieve satisfactory control with twice daily insulin; a few need three or four daily injections.

Practical details regarding the use and adjustment of insulin are not given here because of space limitations, but there is a great deal of information available in *Living with Diabetes: The BDA guide for those treated with insulin* by John Day (see page 87).

VITAL POINT: INSULIN AND TYPE 2 DIABETES

✱ *The decision to change to insulin is a process that may take several months.*

Understanding hyperglycaemia

- Hyperglycaemia is arbitarily defined as a glucose level of > 12 mmol/l.
- It can result from non-compliance with treatment.
- Most patients forget to take their tablets/insulin from time to time. If one dose of tablets/insulin is forgotten within 1 hour of the usual time, take as usual. If longer than this, omit the dose and take the usual dose when the next one is due. DO NOT double the following dose. Accept that blood glucose levels will be temporarily raised.
- Hyperglycaemia may be caused by:
  - untreated diabetes
  - too much food
  - the wrong type of food
  - infections/illness
  - insufficient tablets or insulin (incorrect dose)
  - overuse of particular injection sites – leading to fatty lumps
  - poor injection technique
  - reduction of activity
  - an increase in drugs affecting glycaemic control (e.g. steroid therapy)
  - stress – life changes (retirement, bereavement)
  - weight increase.

Targets for metabolic and risk factor control

	Good	Borderline	Poor
Plasma glucose (mmol/l)			
Fasting	4.4–6.1	6.2–7.8	> 7.8
Postprandial	4.4–8.0	8.1–10.0	> 10.0
HbA1c (%)*	< 7.0	7.0–8.0	> 8.0
Urine glucose (%)	0	0–0.5	> 0.5
Total cholesterol (mmol/l)	< 5.2	5.2–6.5	> 6.5
HDL-cholesterol (mmol/l)	> 1.1	0.9–1.1	< 0.9
Fasting triglycerides (mmol/l)	< 1.7	1.7–2.2	> 2.2
Body mass index (kg/m^2)			
Males	20–25	26–27	> 27
Females	19–24	25–26	> 26
Blood pressure (mmHg)	<130/80	130/80–160/95	> 160/95
Smoking	Non-smoker		Cigarettes

* May vary, depending on local laboratory
References: UKPDS, HOT

Monitoring: the primary care team

- People with diabetes should become accustomed to monitoring their own health, provided that they are capable. You will need to support and check their self-monitoring with them.

- Patients should monitor their own general health and well-being, diabetes control, eyesight, weight, dental care, care of the feet and footwear.

- To promote health and reduce risks of complications, you should teach them how to monitor their diabetes control (urine/blood glucose levels).

- This monitoring allows them to check their own control, take responsibility for their condition and as far as possible maintain independence.

- If you suspect that the person with diabetes has hypoglycaemia (from discussion of symptoms or reports of 'dizzy spells'), blood glucose levels should be checked and medication or insulin reduced.

- Hyperglycaemic episodes will need an increase in tablets or insulin.

- You will have to decide with the patient whether any change in therapy is needed, e.g. diet alone to tablet therapy to combination tablet therapy to combination tablet + insulin therapy to insulin therapy - all in association with dietary guidelines.
- Decisions about adding tablets or insulin should be taken in consultation with the doctor and the person with diabetes.
- By monitoring dietary habits, changes in weight, lifestyle and other medical problems (particularly in elderly people), you can decide when possible review and changes in treatment are necessary.

VITAL POINTS: MONITORING

✱ *It is important that people with diabetes are taught how to monitor their own diabetes.*

✱ *Persistent hyperglycaemia points to the need for a change in therapy.*

Patient and carer information: monitoring your diabetes

General

- Occasional high sugar tests (hyperglycaemia) can be ignored.
- You should look out for the symptoms of hyperglycaemia: thirst; passing urine frequently, particularly at night; lethargy; irritability; blurred vision.
- Persistent hyperglycaemia requires adjustment of food, activity, medication and/or insulin.
- If you are ill or have an infection, your blood sugar (glucose) is likely to climb. If so, contact your GP or care team.
- If you are ill and vomiting, treat this as a medical emergency and summon urgent help.

Urine testing

- Urine testing is important and gives you information about your sugar (glucose) levels.
- If you are unsure of how this is done, then ask at your surgery.
- Urine testing is inexpensive.
- You can get urine testing strips on prescription. You will have to pay for these if you are treated by diet alone.
- Testing and recording your sugar levels helps you control your diabetes.
- Testing a freshly passed urine specimen before breakfast (but not the first one of the day) indicates whether control is good.
- Testing about 2 hours after a meal indicates your highest urinary sugar (glucose) levels.
- Aim at negative urine tests first thing in the morning and 0–1% after food.
- You need a watch or clock with a second hand for home urine testing.
- You should be taught how to record tests and be provided with a testing diary (available free) – ask your care team.

Blood testing

- Confirmation of improved blood sugar (glucose) levels will encourage you to continue with your self-care, treatment and monitoring.
- Blood glucose levels will improve if you can lose weight.
- Many people on tablets for their diabetes like to test their blood glucose for information about their own diabetes, particularly if they suspect hypos or have high blood glucose levels.
- It is important to keep records of all your results. Only in this way will you be able to detect patterns of blood glucose levels that may require a change in medication.

If you have type 2 diabetes and are on tablets or insulin, you are exempt from prescription charges.

Understanding hypoglycaemia

- Hypoglycaemia means a blood glucose level < 3.5 mmol/l.
- Symptoms of hypoglycaemia may be experienced at levels > 3.5 mmol/l, when blood glucose levels have been high over a long period of time (e.g. immediately after diagnosis). This is temporary and will disappear once blood glucose levels settle.
- Hypoglycaemia is more likely to occur in those who have strict control of their blood glucose levels.
- Hypoglycaemia is more common soon after starting a sulphonylurea.
- In elderly people, hypoglycaemia resulting from sulphonylureas carries a high mortality. Consider hospitalisation.
- If the patient is on tablets and has problems with hypoglycaemia, consider a change to a thiazolidinedione or postprandial glucose regulator.

Monitoring: the primary care team

- Hypoglycaemia may occur several hours after extra activity.
- Hypoglycaemia may be caused by:
  - too little food (especially in elderly people);
  - delayed or missed meals;
  - increased medication or insulin;
  - increased activity (exercise);
  - increased mobility;
  - a decrease in concurrent medication affecting glycaemic control;
  - a decrease in weight (particularly in elderly people);
  - the presence of renal failure.

Prevention of hypoglycaemia

- Exercise, alcohol and sexual activity may lower blood sugar (glucose) levels sufficiently to cause hypoglycaemia.
- Eat regularly (meals and snacks).
- Do not delay or miss meals.
- Make sure you have a healthy diet – check with the dietitian.
- Remember to take recommended dose of medication.
- Eat more starchy food if you increase your activity.
- Anyone taking insulin should reduce the dose before strenuous activity.
- Carry glucose tablets/sweets – always (keep in car – if driving).

CARRY IDENTIFICATION (NECKLACE, BRACELET OR CARD)

Treatment of hypoglycaemia

- Recognise symptoms (sweating, trembling, confusion, etc.), which may be special for you.
- Take 4–6 glucose tablets/sweet drink/sweets.
- Follow-up with substantial snack/meal.
- If driving – slow down, stop car safely – remove keys from ignition – move to passenger seat – treat as above.
- Try to work out the cause of this hypoglycaemic attack:
  ? too much insulin;
  ? too little food;
  ? delayed meal;
  ? more activity;
  ? stress;
  ? hot weather;
  ? new injection site used.
  Note: there may be occasions when there is no apparent reason.

5 How to reduce long-term complications of diabetes

Heart & major vessel disease among people with diabetes

- Coronary heart disease (CHD) is much more common among people with diabetes and is the main cause of death (up to 75% in type 2 diabetes).
- The excess risk applies even to those with marginally elevated blood glucose levels, that is > 6 mmol/l.
- Type 2 diabetes increases the risk of myocardial infarct (MI) by two to three times.
- The cardiac risk factors are cumulative.
- Tight control of diabetes and blood pressure reduces the risk of CHD.
- Patients with diabetes should stop smoking.
- Maintain a high index of suspicion for cardiac disease in people with diabetes, even when they have no classic symptoms.
- People with diabetes should have their cholesterol screened on diagnosis. If levels are abnormal (> 5.5 mmol/l), action should be taken; if normal, cholesterol levels should be monitored every 3 years.

Stroke

- Stroke is more frequent in people with diabetes.
- Multi-infarct dementia is also relatively common.
- Prolonged or frequent hypoglycaemia can cause confusion, memory defects or paranoia in older people with diabetes, and may be confused with a stroke or cerebrovascular disease.

Lipids/cholesterol

- Targets: to keep low-density lipoprotein (LDL) cholesterol < 3.5 mmol/l, high-density lipoprotein (HDL) cholesterol > 1.0 mmol/l.
- Treat people with diabetes the same as other patients with known vascular disease.
- Screen all those with diabetes on diagnosis, to achieve optimal control; if control ever deteriorates or insulin is started, they should be screened again. The most reliable test is of fasting glucose levels.
- Treatment is with fibrates, especially if triglycerides are also raised. Statins are a good alternative – and some members of this class are recognised to lower triglycerides as well as cholesterol.
- Those with cardiovascular disease and a cholesterol level of > 5.5 mmol/l should be treated as a secondary prevention patient.
- LDL is an important risk factor. Aim to lower this.
- HDL is also an important risk factor. Aim to raise this if possible.
- TC:HDL (total cholesterol to HDL ratio) is the best lipid marker of cardiovascular risk.
- If raised, a 25% reduction in total cholesterol is a realistic target resulting in significant risk reduction.

Patient and carer information: looking after your heart

- **Diabetes increases the risk of a heart attack.**
- **You should not smoke.**
- **You should eat healthily and see a dietitian to check this out.**
- **You should have your cholesterol checked on diagnosis of your diabetes.**
- **You should have your cholesterol/lipids measured at least every 3 years.**
- **You should have regular blood pressure measurements and be prepared to start treatment if it is raised.**
- **Go to your GP if you have any pain in your chest, arm or jaw, or have pain when exercising.**
- **Good control of blood sugar (glucose) reduces the risk of heart disease and stroke.**

Feet

Peripheral vascular disease

* People with diabetes are 2–4 times more likely to develop intermittent claudication and 4–6 times more likely to have to undergo an amputation.
* Screen all people with diabetes for peripheral vascular disease.
* Ask about their smoking history and symptoms of intermittent claudication.
* After 20 years of diabetes, 50% of men and 33% of women have no pulses in their feet.
* At annual review, check patients' feet for ischaemia and feel for the pulses.
* Refer any patients with gradually worsening symptoms or rest pain to a vascular surgeon.
* Transfer any patients with critical ischaemia or gangrene to hospital immediately.

VITAL POINT: LONG-TERM COMPLICATIONS

✱ *Raised blood glucose and blood pressure are major risk factors for heart disease, stroke and peripheral circulatory problems.*

Peripheral neuropathy

* Evidence of neuropathy may be found in up to 50% of patients with type 2 diabetes, causing problems for about one-third of them.
* Peripheral neuropathy affects 50% of people with diabetes.
* Lower limb and foot problems caused by peripheral neuropathy and ischaemia are common, causing prolonged hospital admission and amputation.
* Identification of those at risk of foot ulceration and educating these patients are important preventive measures.

Monitoring: the primary care team

Examination of the feet

With a little practice, a thorough foot examination can be carried out in a few minutes. All people with diabetes should have access to a state-registered podiatrist. If there are any concerns, make a referral.

- Remove shoes, socks (tights or stockings).
- Examine the patient lying on a couch or seated comfortably with both legs and feet raised.
- Examine both feet for the following:
  - condition of the skin (lower legs and feet);
  - dry, flaky skin;
  - cracks or evidence of fungal infection between each toe (athlete's foot);
  - colour of skin (lower legs and feet);
  - corns, calluses, other deformities (on pressure-bearing points, e.g. tops of toes);
  - condition of toe nails (whether thickened, long or horny);
  - nail-cutting technique/ingrowing toe nails;
  - discoloration/abnormal skin lesions;
  - evidence of infection, i.e. pain, lack of sensation, numbness, inflammation, cellulitis, exudate or swelling.
- Examine upper, lower surfaces of feet and toes (including heels) carefully.
- Record all abnormalities/changes.
- Examine the feet for the following:
  - dorsalis pedis and posterior tibial pulses;
  - if foot pulses are diminished, palpate popliteal and femoral pulses;
  - record changed, diminished or absent pulses;
  - sensation testing – check pressure using a 10 g monofilament, check vibration perception using a 128-Hz tuning fork and test from toe to mid-calf region;
  - for comparison, the stimulus should first be applied to the patient's outstretched arm and then repeated on the lower limbs and feet – with the eyes closed;

- test for motor neuropathy by looking for deformities in the toes and feet;
- check knee and ankle jerks (with a tendon hammer);
- record defects in sensation;
- examine foot ulcers for inflammation and discharge (take swab for bacterial analysis);
- record and discuss foot problems with the patient as appropriate.

Examination of the shoes

Shoes should be examined inside and outside, looking for evidence of the following:

- General wear and tear.
- The need for repair.
- Gait change (one shoe more worn than the other).
- Excessive weight bearing (heel on sole worn down).
- Perforation of soles or heels (by nails, etc.).
- Abrasive heels (especially with new shoes).
- Damaging projections inside the shoes (causing pressure).
- Worn insoles (causing pressure).
- Poor fit of shoes (length and breadth).

Problems identified with shoes should be recorded and discussed with the patient.

Examination of socks/tights/stockings

Socks, tight or stocking should be examined for:

- Type of material (whether constricting – nylon or elasticated).
- Type of washing powder used (biological washing powders can be irritant).
- Method of holding up socks (e.g. garters should not be used).
- Presence and thickness of seams (these can cause traumatic ulcers).

Problems identified should be recorded and discussed with the patient.

People at risk

* People who live alone.
* Those who drink too much alcohol.
* Those with poor eye sight.
* Those with poor glycaemic control.
* Those with a poor self-image.
* Those who live in deprived areas.
* Those with other complications of diabetes.
* Those who smoke.
* Male sex.
* Those who walk or climb in footwear seldom worn, or those who enjoy walking bare foot.

VITAL POINTS: FEET

✱ Emphasise to smokers that, as well as the better known consequences of smoking, they are also putting their feet at risk.

✱ Examine the feet at least once a year.

✱ Examine the feet to educate yourself and your patient.

✱ Failure to do this may result in unnecessary amputations.

Patient and carer information: looking after your feet

- Keep your feet clean: wash and dry gently between your toes.
- Moisturise your feet with hand cream, olive oil or E45 cream, but not between your toes.
- Do not dig down the sides of your toenails.
- Cut your nails (softer after washing) according to the shape of your toes. If you cannot cut your own then request a visit to a state-registered chiropodist (podiatrist).
- Check your feet and shoes daily – using a mirror if necessary. You may not be aware of injury.
- If possible involve a third party, such as your partner.
- Do not ignore even the slightest injury to your feet.
- Report any sores, swelling, cracks, corns, skin damage or change of colour IMMEDIATELY to your doctor.
- Avoid walking barefoot; you should wear shoes or slippers at all times.
- Choose shoes that provide good support: broad, long and deep. Check that you can wriggle your toes inside your shoes. As a general rule trainers are a good choice.
- Try to buy shoes where you can have them fitted by a trained person.
- Wear new shoes for short periods of time to start with.
- Check your shoes regularly for ridges, sharp points or nails; tip them out upside down before putting on.
- Wear the correct shoes for the job and for the health of your feet.
- Do not wear tight-fitting socks; choose ones with no ridges but if they have them wear socks inside out; change daily.
- Avoid extremes of temperature, very hot baths, sitting close to fires and radiators, and hot water bottles.
- Do not treat corns yourself; visit a state-registered chiropodist.
- Never use a surgical blade, corn-paring knife or corn remedies on your feet.
- Treat your feet with respect.

Diabetic retinopathy

Monitoring: the primary care team

- Check that an optician is being visited annually for visual acuity checks.
- Arrange retinal screening programmes, whether with photography and/or an accredited optometrist as locally available.
- If diabetic retinopathy is detected:
  - support the person sympathetically;
  - give information about the extent of retinal damage, and
  - if sight threatening, ensure that the person is referred immediately to an ophthalmologist;
  - give support and reassurance because the individual will fear possible visual loss and treatment; there may be a bad family history of diabetic eye disease.
- Give information about laser therapy if required.
- As chronic glaucoma is more common in people with diabetes, ensure that intraocular pressure is measured every year.
- Ensure appropriate and timely referral to an ophthalmologist.
- People with diabetes are more likely to develop cataracts; these must be treated early to allow the early detection of retinopathy. Arrange for an ophthalmological referral, so that cataract extraction can be undertaken as soon as appropriate (a waiting list priority).

VITAL POINT: EYES

* *Ensure that all patients with type 2 diabetes have their retinas checked or photographed by someone competent every year.*

Patient and carer information: looking after your eyes

General

- You must have your eyes checked once a year with eye drops, either using a retinal camera or by someone expert in examining the retina (back of the eye).

- You are entitled to a free annual eye test if you take tablets or insulin, so use this facility.

- Ask your care team to explain what is being checked and what is happening.

- If, on examination, you are found to have a condition called diabetic retinopathy, you will be referred to an ophthalmologist and possibly for laser therapy.

- If you need laser therapy, ask for an information sheet about it.

- Laser treatment may not improve your sight; it prevents further deterioration.

Laser therapy

- Laser therapy is given to prevent the progress of diabetic disease at the back of the eye (retina).

- Ideally, you should be given laser therapy at an early stage <u>before</u> your sight has been affected. Regular eye screening is important.

- The laser is a machine that produces a small spot of very bright light.

- The light is so bright it produces a burn wherever it is focused.

- Although the laser makes a burn in your eye, it is not usually painful because the retina cannot feel pain.

- Sometimes, however, if you have had a lot of laser treatment, it may be uncomfortable and you will be offered a local anaesthetic.

- Laser treatment is usually carried out in an outpatient department.

- You will be able to go home after the treatment.

- Your vision may be blurred or you may be dazzled by bright light (take dark glasses with you).

- You should not drive home after laser therapy.

- It is best to be accompanied to the laser clinic.

- After the treatment, you may notice some reduction in your sight. This usually only lasts a few days. You may experience headaches.

- As only one eye is treated at a time, if your other eye sees well, your vision should not be too badly affected.

- Most people do not need to take time off work after treatment.
- You are required to declare on your driving licence application form that you have had laser treatment. You will probably need a visual fields test (to test the extent of your vision).
- If you need large amounts of laser treatment, your field of vision may be affected.
- Provided that you can read a number plate at 20.5 metres (67 feet) with or without spectacles, and you pass the visual fields test, as most people do, there will be no problem about your driving licence. You will need to adhere to the usual regulations for someone with diabetes.

Diabetic nephropathy

Monitoring: the primary care team

- Up to 40% of people with type 2 diabetes have some degree of kidney disease.
- There are four stages of diabetic renal disease:
  - stage 1 or microalbuminuria: urine needs to be sent to the laboratory to detect microalbuminuria;
  - stage 2 or albuminuria: detected in the clinic using a semi-quantitative dipstick;
  - stage 3 or raised serum creatinine: once this is above the normal range, over half the normal kidney function has been lost;
  - stage 4 or end-stage renal failure, requiring dialysis.
- Delaying the progression of diabetic nephropathy involves three separate actions:
  - aggressive control of blood pressure, which is nearly always raised;
  - tight blood glucose control;
  - in type 1 diabetes, dietary protein restriction may be of benefit.
- Established renal failure will require the following treatment options:
  - haemodialysis;
  - continuous ambulatory peritoneal dialysis (CAPD);
  - renal transplantation.
- Monitor renal function over the first 2 months of starting patients on ACE inhibitors.

VITAL POINT: KIDNEYS

*** Treat raised BP very aggressively in patients with kidney disease. This will postpone end-stage renal failure.**

Autonomic neuropathy and sexual dysfunction

Monitoring: the primary care team

Autonomic neuropathy affects 20–40% of all people with diabetes.

It may contribute to impotence in up to 50% of men with long-standing diabetes. Treatment for this condition is available.

- This is often a 'hidden' problem.
- May be the cause of marital difficulties.
- Failure to gain an erection may be caused by:
    - nerve damage;
    - poor circulation;
    - psychological factors;
    - drinking alcohol, smoking and recreational drugs, and treatment for BP and depression.
- Treatment is available and is offered after assessment for possible causes. Treatments currently considered/offered are:
    - counselling;
    - vacuum devices;
    - self-injection of alprostadil (Caverject, Viridal) into the penis;
    - penile implants (surgery);
    - sildenafil (Viagra): this is available in limited quantities to men with diabetes and erection difficulties. It is safe but should never be used by men taking a nitrate for their heart, which includes glyceryl trinitrate (GTN) tablets or spray for angina.
- Referral is recommended.

Patient and carer information: sexual issues

- Alcohol, smoking, recreational drugs and medication (for blood pressure or depression) can cause problems with erection.
- You will have blood tests to check your diabetes control and hormone levels.
- You could be referred to a specialist clinic.
- There are various effective treatments: counselling, injections, vacuum devices, surgery, tablets.
- The drug Viagra (sildenafil) can be obtained in limited supplies. Do not use if you are taking a nitrate for your heart.

Impact of the menopause: recommendations

- Postmenopausal women who have diabetes may be advised to take hormone replacement therapy (HRT) because this can help to protect against heart disease and osteoporosis.
- Women can try different types of HRT until a suitable one is found.
- HRT can increase breast cancer risk in some women so they will need to take part in a screening programme, as should all women over 50 according to national guidelines.
- For women who also take insulin, starting HRT may require a small dose adjustment.

6 How to manage type 1 diabetes

Type 1 diabetes (insulin-dependent diabetes or IDDM): presentation and diagnosis

- Diabetes care is a partnership between patients and professionals. However, at the onset, many patients will want the doctor and nurse to assume control. With time, patients gain in confidence and ownership of their diabetes.

- Most people with type 1 diabetes are seen by a diabetes care team in secondary care, although they will occasionally present to the surgery.

- Treat with insulin. Options for different insulin regimens should be discussed regularly. For up-to-date information, refer to British National Formulary or MIMS.

- Basic lifestyle advice, such as NOT SMOKING, reduces the risks of heart disease, stroke and poor circulation.

- People with type 1 diabetes feel more confident if they monitor their blood glucose levels several times a day, understand the results and take action on them.

- The purpose of the monitoring is good glucose control, to keep people feeling well and to help to avoid both high and low blood glucose levels.

- A range of blood glucose levels needs to be discussed. The ideal is 4–7 mmol/l before and < 10 mmol/l after a meal.

- They must be aware of possible short- and long-term complications of their diabetes.

- Regular visits and checks throughout the year provide opportunities for discussion and/or advice.

- People with diabetes should expect an annual review: eye check with drops, foot inspection, blood pressure, urine albumin.

- Advise that there can also be problems with good glucose control: weight gain, more severe hypos and less warning of a hypo. Help should be requested if any of these occur.

- People with diabetes need to find their own way of coping with diabetes in a way that suits their lifestyle.

Children and young people: main issues

- A child presenting with symptoms of diabetes needs immediate referral to hospital or a specialist diabetes centre for confirmation of diagnosis and assessment.
- The management plan should involve the primary care team.
- The primary health care team must be kept advised of the child's health by the specialist team.
- You need to be prepared to talk with the child and family.
- Such children should receive the usual immunisations.
- Children with diabetes often have large fluctuations in their glucose control (especially if ill) and the primary care team need to be able to deal with this.
- When these children come to the surgery with other ailments, these should be considered in the light of their diabetes.
- You should be available to provide extra support to the child and the family at difficult times such as changing school, puberty, etc.
- The family may well need considerably more support than the average family.
- Observe carefully relationships within the family and be prepared to address these directly with the parents.

VITAL POINT: TYPE 1 DIABETES

* Make friends with your patients, and help them accept their diabetes.

7 How to manage pregnancy and gestational diabetes

Pregnant women with diabetes

- Any woman with diabetes contemplating pregnancy must have pre-pregnancy counselling with her partner.
- All women planning a pregnancy should take folic acid.
- Pregnancy complicates diabetes and diabetes complicates pregnancy.
- Blood glucose control needs to be optimised (levels between 4 and 7 mmol/l) before and throughout pregnancy to prevent complications/abnormalities in the baby and complications in the mother.
- The woman needs to be aware of the risk of congenital abnormalities.
- The risks to the woman are: retinopathy can worsen and kidney damage may increase.
- The aim is normal delivery of baby but caesarean section is more likely (50% have this) if glucose control is poor.
- Drugs cannot be used in pregnancy so control has to be by diet and insulin. Those with type 2 diabetes have to start insulin, as drugs may cause danger to the unborn baby.
- A planned programme of care, with precise protocols, should be available to all the care teams and the mother.
- Optimal blood glucose control increases the risk of hypoglycaemia.
- Blood glucose should be monitored four to six times a day.
- Insulin will need adjusting, often reaching two to three times the non-pregnant dose.
- Diet should be controlled, with care about food intake and weight.
- Overall good nutrition is essential.
- Access to specialist nurses and midwives is necessary.
- All women with diabetes must visit the diabetic clinic at least every 4 weeks: HbAlc, blood pressure and urine albumin tested every visit; eyes checked regularly; scans as agreed locally.
- A planned delivery programme is needed.

Gestational diabetes mellitus (GDM)

- This is diabetes that starts/occurs only during pregnancy.
- If fasting blood glucose is borderline, you must confirm the diagnosis by an oral glucose tolerance test.
- Most antenatal services have protocols for identifying GDM.
- Referral to a specialist diabetes team is recommended.
- If diabetes presents late in pregnancy, it has probably been hidden throughout the pregnancy. Urgent referral required.
- Pregnant women have a lower renal threshold so glycosuria is not diagnostic of gestational diabetes.
- Management is by diet and monitoring of weight.
- Drugs are not used.
- If blood glucose levels are not kept within range by diet (< 6 mmol/l before meals and < 9 mmol/l after), then you need to start insulin.
- Frequent blood glucose monitoring is necessary.
- Women should have blood glucose check at 6-week postnatal visit, by which time levels should have returned to normal, although they are more likely to have IGT or IFG.
- Of those who develop gestational diabetes, 40% will develop type 2 diabetes later in life.
- Women who have gestational diabetes need to be informed of this problem and counselled about maintaining a healthy lifestyle to reduce the risk of type 2 diabetes: plenty of exercise and weight control.

VITAL POINTS: PREGNANCY AND DIABETES

✳ Early referral to obstetric diabetes service is essential.

✳ 40% of women with gestational diabetes will develop type 2 diabetes in later life.

Patient and carer information: living with diabetes

Living with diabetes means looking after yourself – not just the control of blood sugar (glucose), but also your feet, eyes, teeth (dentist) and making sure you are up to date with your immunisations. In other words it is looking after your health generally. There are also certain areas where you will have to be particularly careful (such as family planning or travelling), or be aware of possible legal restrictions (such as driving).

Immunisation

- All the normal immunisations recommended are safe for you.
- If you are travelling abroad check with your GP whether any further immunisations are needed.
- If you are aged over 65, and provided that it will not cause a problem for you, you are entitled to a 'flu immunisation: this is usually available during October/November each year.
- Pneumococcal immunisation is available to anyone over 2 years of age with diabetes; it can be given with the influenza immunisation.
- Immunisation can have an effect on your diabetes; test your sugar (glucose) levels more frequently and if necessary increase your dose of insulin or tablets.

Dental care

- Your dentist should be informed of your diabetes.
- Go for regular check-ups.
- Get early treatment because infections can upset your sugar (glucose) control.
- General anaesthetics should be carried out in hospital.
- A painful mouth can cause low blood sugar (glucose) levels if eating becomes difficult.
- You will not receive any special financial help with dental fees.

Family planning advice (for women)

- Ask for advice about pregnancy well before you plan to have children.
- The contraceptive pill does not suit everybody. It may carry extra risks if you are older, overweight or smoke, or if you have high blood pressure or a tendency to blood clots.
- Low-dose combined contraceptive pills do not usually have any effects on diabetes, but you should check your blood sugar (glucose) levels and have regular blood pressure tests.
- Low-dose progestogen-only pills are safe in diabetes, but are less reliable than the low-dose combined pill.
- You can use the coil (IUD) or barrier methods (caps and condoms); you can be sterilised and your partner can have a vasectomy.

Patient and carer information: living with diabetes

Driving

- Car driving licences can be held by people with diabetes.

- Licences are renewed every one, two or three years depending on health (of people treated with insulin).

- Those treated with diet alone or tablets are not subject to licence restrictions (for diabetes). They can retain their 'until aged 70' privilege, but must inform the DVLA if there is any change to treatment.

- The DVLA (tel: 01792 772151) must be told of your diabetes and any treatment change (e.g. from diet alone to tablets or tablets to insulin), except if the diabetes is diet controlled. This is required by law.

  Note: this information must be provided and recorded. The decision to follow this advice is the responsibility of the individual concerned.

- Licence renewal forms are sent automatically before the expiry date. There is no fee for renewal.

- Licence renewal is granted after completion of the form by the person with diabetes (including signed consent for the individual's doctor to be consulted by the DVLA, if required).

- A medical check may be requested by the DVLA.

- The driver must inform his or her driving insurance company of the presence of diabetes.

- Some insurance companies load the driver's premium. This should be challenged. It is sensible to 'shop around' because the Disability Discrimination Act 1995 has improved this situation. Diabetes UK Trading can also offer motor insurance cover (Motor Quoteline: 0800 731 7432).

Travelling abroad

- You may require immunisation, which could affect your blood sugar (glucose) control.
- Travel insurance needs to include adequate cover, including for your diabetes; contact Diabetes UK for information (tel: 0800 731 7431).
- Obtain form E111 from your surgery or local DSS office, which provides information on travelling and health, and medical care in the European Community.
- Take with you: identification; doctor's letter; medication for travel sickness and diarrhoea; antibiotics; simple dressings; supply of diabetes medication; protection against sun burn; appropriate footwear; and sweets or biscuits for travel. Take testing equipment and cool bag if treated with insulin; keep supplies in a cool bag and carry in hand luggage.

Life insurance

- Life insurance is calculated according to age and state of health and likelihood of survival
- A life insurance policy already held should not be affected by the diagnosis of diabetes. It is not necessary to declare your diabetes once a policy has been agreed.
- If a new policy is taken out, your diabetes must be declared and the policy may be loaded. This can be challenged.
- Advice about sympathetic insurance companies can be obtained from Diabetes UK (tel: 0800 731 7433).

9 Emergencies and illness

Emergencies

Action: the primary care team

IMMEDIATE REFERRAL TO HOSPITAL:

- Person with severe hypoglycaemia not responding to glucagon.
- Person with severe ketosis/ketoacidosis.
- Newly diagnosed person with type 1 diabetes and severe symptoms.
- Newly diagnosed person with type 2 diabetes and severe symptoms.
- Child diagnosed with diabetes and severe symptoms.
- Person with diabetes who is severely dehydrated (hyperosmolar coma), particularly older people.
- Sudden deterioration in foot ulcer (e.g. any change in colour, new onset of pain, redness or swelling).
- Sudden deterioration in sight (e.g. retinal haemorrage/retinal detachment).

Ketoacidosis

- If ketoacidosis develops, refer straight to hospital. Start treatment straightaway.
- Intravenous fluids are needed.
- Blood glucose levels should be closely monitored.
- Death in these patients may be the result of delay in treatment.
- Ketoacidosis is the most common cause of death in people with diabetes aged under 20.
- The most common causes of severe ketoacidosis remain delay in diagnosing type 1 and wrong advice given (incorrect instructions to stop insulin during intercurrent illness). Correct advice is to keep testing blood glucose and taking insulin, which usually need to be increased, depending on the results.

VITAL POINT: EMERGENCIES

✱ Patients on insulin should keep taking their insulin during illness.

Illness

Action: the primary care team

- Monitoring equipment such as Ketostix and blood glucose test strips (in date and kept in airtight containers in a dry place, not in a fridge) should be available in the surgery and doctor's bag.
- Short-acting insulin may be useful to lower blood glucose levels in acute illness (in surgery and doctor's bag).
- Review therapy and treat intercurrent illness.
- Consider short-term insulin therapy.
- Vomiting/hyperglycaemia/ketosis is a medical emergency and requires hospital admission for intravenous insulin and fluids.
- Blood glucose control may deteriorate rapidly during an illness of any kind. Teach people with diabetes when they need to get help.
- Also teach the relative or carer in case the person with diabetes is too unwell to behave rationally.
- For those with type 2 diabetes and who are on insulin, if it is possible and appropriate, teach the relative or carer to draw up and give insulin if necessary and be able to monitor blood or urine glucose levels.
- Give an emergency contact telephone number to the person with diabetes or a relative.
- Glucagon for treatment of severe hypoglycaemia.

VITAL POINT: ILLNESS

✱ For people with diabetes, vomiting is a danger sign and needs urgent action.

Patient and carer information: what to do when you're ill

- A minor illness, such as a cold, may cause your blood sugar (glucose) levels to rise.
- Keep taking your tablets (or insulin) even if you are not eating.
- Blood glucose levels will return to normal once the infection is over.
- Consult your doctor if the illness persists, if you have symptoms of high glucose levels or if you have high test results.
- Headaches and sore throats can be safely treated with paracetamol or aspirin.
- Sugar-free cough remedies are available from your local pharmacist.
- Vomiting may prevent you keeping down tablets – consult your doctor.
- Vomiting and diarrhoea may cause serious loss of fluid – consult your doctor.
- You may need this fluid replaced by means of a drip.
- You may need insulin for a short time.

IMPORTANT RULES

- Continue with your diabetes treatment (diet and tablets or insulin).
- Ensure that you drink plenty of liquid (water, tea, etc.).
- Test urine or blood every day to check on how you are doing.
- If you are not hungry, substitute meals with a liquid or light diet (soup, ice cream, glucose drinks, milk).
- Consult your doctor in good time.

10 Monitoring care in the practice

Practice and shared protocols

- Need ongoing clinical audit of practice-based diabetes services.
- Select the criteria for audit.
- Agree standards of care for audit.
- MAAGs (Medical Audit Advisory Groups) can be of help in facilitating clinical audit.
- Anonymous data from district, regional and national groups enable evaluation of effectiveness.
- St Vincent's declaration sets out targets for improving outcome in the long term.
- In the short term, monitor: process of care, prevalence of cardiovascular risk factors and markers of late complications, and acute and intermediate outcomes.
- It is valuable to collate data at a district level on a district diabetes register.

Audit and quality control monitoring

Process measures

- Prevalence of diagnosed diabetes.
- Proportion of patients who have had annual review:
  - BMI;
  - dietary advice by dietitian;
  - smoking;
  - urinalysis for proteinuria, including microalbuminuria screening, albumin excretion;
  - blood pressure;
  - HbAlc;
  - serum lipids (HDL:LDL);

- serum creatinine;
- eyes: visual acuity and fundoscopy;
- feet and footwear: evidence of circulation problems and neuropathy.
• Patient satisfaction: questionnaire.

Outcome measures

• Health status and quality of life: psychological and physical well-being; knowledge of diabetes, self-care performance.
• Glycaemic control:
  - patients with HbA1c > 7.0%;
  - patients needing hospital admission for ketoacidosis;
  - patients needing professional attention for hypoglycaemia.
• Prevalence of cardiovascular risk factors
  - patients who smoke;
  - BMI > 25;
  - patients taking no regular physical activity;
  - patients with BP > 130/80;
  - patients with raised cholesterol (> 5.2 mmol/l);
  - patients with raised triglycerides (>1.7 mmol/l).
• Markers of microvascular risk factors:
  - patients with proteinuria/microalbuminuria;
  - patients with raised creatinine (above normal range);
  - patients who needed laser therapy/vitrectomy for diabetic retinopathy;
  - patients with background and sight-threatening retinopathy;
  - patients with absent foot pulses;
  - patients with reduced vibration sense;
  - patients with foot ulceration (previous or present).
• Intermediate outcomes:
  - patients with cataract;
  - patients with angina;
  - patients with claudication;
  - patients with symptomatic neuropathy;
  - male patients with erectile dysfunction.

- Outcomes of pregnancies in women presenting with pre-existing or gestational diabetes:
  - birth rates;
  - abortion rates: spontaneous and terminations;
  - stillbirth rates and peri-/neonatal mortality rates;
  - incidence of congenital abnormalities.
- Late outcomes:
  - patients who have had myocardial infarction;
  - patients who have had a stroke;
  - patients with visual impairment;
  - patients with end-stage renal failure;
  - patients who have had above- or below-ankle amputation;
  - age-specific mortality in people with diabetes.

These recommendations are from the Diabetes UK document – see resources list on page 87.

Glossary of terms

ACE inhibitor: a class of drugs whose names end in 'pril', used in hypertension and cardiac failure. They are thought to protect the kidneys in early nephropathy.

albuminuria: the presence of albumin in the urine may denote a urinary infection or early kidney damage.

autonomic neuropathy: damage to the system of nerves that regulate many autonomic functions of the body such as stomach emptying, sexual function (potency) and blood pressure control.

beta blockers: drugs that block the effect of stress hormones on the cardiovascular system. Often used to treat angina and raised blood pressure. Change the warning signs of hypoglycaemia.

beta cell (β cell): the cell that produces insulin, found in the islets of Langerhans in the pancreas.

biguanides: a group of tablets that lower blood glucose levels. The only one in use is metformin.

blood glucose monitoring: system of measuring blood glucose levels at home using special reagent sticks or a special meter.

body mass index (BMI): body weight corrected for height expressed as weight in kg/(height in metres)^2. Normal 20-25 kg/m^2.

diabetes mellitus: a disorder of the pancreas characterised by a high blood glucose level.

Diabetes UK: formerly known as the British Diabetic Association (BDA). Founded in 1938 by RD Lawrence, the foremost doctor specialising in diabetes, and HG Wells, the famous author. Both had diabetes and Diabetes UK has maintained the positive collaboration between people with diabetes and health care professionals.

diabetic coma: extreme form of hyperglycaemia, usually with ketoacidosis, causing unconsciousness.

diabetic nephropathy: kidney damage caused by diabetes.

diabetic neuropathy: nerve damage caused by diabetes.

diabetic retinopathy: retinal damage caused by diabetes.

dietary fibre: part of plant material that resists digestion and gives bulk to the diet. Also called fibre or roughage.

diuretics: drugs that increase the volume of urine, usually called water tablets.

fructosamine: measurement of glucose control, similar to HbA1c; it reflects average blood sugar (glucose) over previous 2–3 weeks. Cheaper but less reliable than HbA1c.

gestational diabetes mellitus (GDM): diabetes occurring during pregnancy with recovery after delivery.

glaucoma: disease of the eye causing increased pressure inside the eyeball.

glitazones: drugs (also called thiazolidinediones or PPAR-gamma agonists) that reduce blood glucose and insulin levels. This is achieved by an improvement in insulin resistance, resulting in increased effectiveness of available insulin in liver, fat and muscle.

glucose tolerance test: test used in the diagnosis of diabetes. The glucose in the blood is measured before and up to 2 hours after the person has drunk 75 g of glucose while fasting.

glucagon: a hormone which can be injected to increase blood glucose level. Used in severe hypos.

glycosuria: presence of glucose in the urine.

HbA1c (glycated haemoglobin): the part of the haemoglobin that has glucose attached to it. Its measurement is a test of diabetes control. The amount in the blood depends on the average blood glucose level over the previous 2–3 months.

hyperglycaemia: high blood glucose (> 12 mmol/l).

hyperlipidaemia: an excess of fats (or lipids) in the blood.

hypo: abbreviation for hypoglycaemia.

hypoglycaemia (also known as a hypo or an insulin reaction): low blood glucose (< 3.5 mmol/l).

impaired fasting glycaemia (IFG): this is a new category, which includes people with fasting glucose levels above normal, but not enough to diagnose diabetes, i.e. between 6.1 and 7.0 mmol/l

impaired glucose tolerance (IGT): is defined by a 2-hour glucose during an OGTT of > 7.8 mmol/l, but < 11.1 mmol/l or a fasting plasma glucose < 7.0 mmol/l.

insulin resistance: condition in which higher concentrations of insulin are required to achieve the same biological effect.

islets of Langerhans: specialised cells within the pancreas that produce insulin and glucagon.

ketoacidosis: a serious condition caused by lack of insulin and very high blood glucose levels which results in body fat being used up to form ketones and acids. Characterised by high blood glucose levels, ketones in the urine, vomiting, drowsiness, heavy laboured breathing and a smell of acetone on the breath.

ketonuria: the presence of acetone and other ketones in the urine. Detected by testing with a special testing stick (Ketostix, Ketur Test) or tablet (Acetest). Presence of ketones in the urine is due to lack of insulin or periods of starvation.

laser treatment: process in which laser beams are used to treat a damaged retina (back of the eye). Widely used in diabetic retinopathy.

metabolic syndrome: a cluster of medical problems – diabetes, hypertension, central obesity, abnormal lipids, coronary heart disease – all linked to insulin resistance. Also known as insulin resistance syndrome, Reaven's syndrome or syndrome X.

microalbuminuria: excretion of traces of protein in the urine; an indication of early and treatable renal disease. Also a marker of macrovascular complications.

nephropathy: kidney damage. In the first instance this makes the kidney more leaky so that albumin appears in the urine. At a later stage it may affect the function of the kidney and in severe cases lead to kidney failure.

neuropathy: damage to the nerves, which may be peripheral neuropathy or autonomic neuropathy. Occurs in diabetes, especially when poorly controlled.

oral glucose tolerance test (OGTT): blood glucose is measured fasting and after 75 g glucose syrup. The most important value is taken at 2 hours.

peripheral neuropathy: damage to the nerves supplying the muscles and skin. This can result in diminished sensation and/or pain, particularly in the feet and legs, and in muscle weakness.

polydipsia: being excessively thirsty and drinking too much. A symptom of untreated diabetes and high blood glucose levels.

polyuria: the passing of large quantities of urine as a result of excess glucose in the blood stream. A symptom of untreated diabetes and high blood glucose levels.

postprandial glucose regulators: drugs that reduce blood glucose levels. Have a similar mode of action to sulphonylureas, but with a faster onset and shorter duration of action.

PPAR-gamma agonists: drugs (also called thiazolidinediones or glitazones) that reduce blood glucose and insulin levels. This is achieved by an improvement in insulin resistance, resulting in increased effectiveness of available insulin in liver, fat and muscle.

Primary Care Diabetes United Kingdom (PCD UK): a professional section of Diabetes UK, devoted to the interests of primary care, where the vast majority of people with diabetes receive management of their disease.

proteinuria: protein or albumin in the urine.

retinopathy: damage to the retina.

sulphonylureas: tablets that lower the blood glucose by stimulating the pancreas to produce more insulin. Commonly used sulphonylureas are glibenclamide, gliclazide, glipizide and chlorpropamide.

thiazolidinediones: drugs (also called PPAR-gamma agonists or glitazones) that reduce blood glucose and insulin levels. This is achieved by an improvement in insulin resistance, resulting in increased effectiveness of available insulin in liver, fat and muscle.

type 1 diabetes: this type of diabetes refers to young people who usually develop diabetes over a short space of time and always need insulin. Previously called insulin-dependent diabetes (IDDM).

type 2 diabetes: this is the more common form of diabetes, which usually develops in middle age and initially responds to diet and/or tablets. Most people, however, end up needing insulin. Previously called non-insulin-dependent diabetes (NIDDM).

UK Prospective Diabetes Study (UKPDS): a study designed to answer the question of whether tight control of blood glucose and blood pressure influenced the outcome of type 2 diabetes. The results, published in September 1998, suggested that tight control of both factors lead to positive benefits in reducing the risk of diabetic complications.

Resources

Self-help for the primary care team

- Organise your own education by attending courses/conferences.
- Find a 'buddy' practice to befriend and learn and share experiences.
- Locate a 'mentor' practice with long experience of provision of diabetes care.
- Contact the hospital-based local diabetes team and request resources and education.
- Contact Diabetes UK for further information (see page 90).
- Driving and diabetes: see the Diabetes UK leaflet (see page 90).
- Join Diabetes UK (PCDUK).

Mainly for general practitioners

- Postgraduate Course in Diabetes held annually – changing centres every 2–3 years. Details from specialist diabetes physicians or Diabetes UK.
- Local initiatives – through General Practitioner Training Schemes. Postgraduate Centres, RCGP Training, Diabetes Team Initiatives (PGEA schemes usually sought).
- Warwick Diabetes Care (University of Warwick) – a coherent point of contact for all those involved in providing diabetes care in the following ways: providing and promoting multidisciplinary diabetes education courses for health care professionals; undertaking and supporting applied diabetes research; developing practical resources and people networks.

Useful reports/key references

Alberti KGMM (1999). The diagnosis and classification of diabetes mellitus. *Diabetes Voice* 44: 35-41.

Audit Commission National Report (2000). *Test Times - a review of diabetes services in England and Wales.* Oxon: Audit Commission Publications.

British Diabetic Association/Department of Health (1995). *Report of the St Vincent Task Force for Diabetes.* London: BDA.

British Diabetic Association (1995). *Diabetes in the United Kingdom - 1996.* A BDA Report. London: BDA.

British Diabetic Association (1997). *Recommendations for the Management of Diabetes in Primary Care.* London: BDA.

Hansson L *et al.* (1998). The Hypertension Optimal Treatment (HOT) Study: 24 month data on blood pressure and tolerability. *Lancet* 1998; 351: 1755-612.

HMSO (1999). *Saving Lives: Our Healthier Nation.* White Paper, Cm 4386. London: The Stationery Office.

Marks L (1996). *Counting the Cost: The real impact of non-insulin-dependent diabetes.* London: King's Fund/BDA.

Pierce M, Agarwal G, Ridout D (2000). A survey of diabetes care in general practice in England and Wales. *British Journal of General Practice* 2000; 50: 542-5.

Poole Study (1998). Budd S *et al. Diabetic Medicine* 1998 (suppl 2); 511.

Royal College of Physicians/British Diabetic Association (1993). *Good Practice in the Diagnosis and Treatment of NIDDM.* London: RCP/BDA.

UKPDS 33. *Lancet* 1998; 352: 837-53.   UKPDS 36. *BMJ* 2000; 321: 412-19.

UKPDS 34. *Lancet* 1998; 352: 854-65.   UKPDS 38. *BMJ* 1998; 317: 703-13.

UKPDS 35. *BMJ* 2000; 321: 405-12.   UKPDS 39. *BMJ* 1998; 317: 713-20

Useful websites

Diabetes UK: www.diabetes.org.uk

Medscape - an excellent free resource with a section on diabetes: www.medscape.com

British Medical Journal - free access: www.bmj.com

Joslin Diabetes Centre - educational website: www.joslin.harvard.edu/education

Warwick Diabetes Care - www.diabetescare.warwick.ac.uk

Useful books

Alexander WD (1998). *Diabetic Retinopathy: A guide for diabetes care teams*. Oxford: Blackwell Science.

Areffio A, Hill RD, Leigh O (1992). *Diabetes and Primary Eye Care*. Oxford: Blackwell Science.

Campbell IW, Lebovitz H (1996). *Fast Facts - Diabetes Mellitus*. Oxford: Health Press.

Day J (1998). *Living with Diabetes: The BDA guide for those treated with insulin*. Chichester: John Wiley & Sons.

Day J (1998). *Living with Diabetes: The BDA guide for those treated with diet and exercise*. Chichester: John Wiley & Sons.

Dornhorst D, Hadden DR (eds) (1996). *Diabetes and Pregnancy. An international approach to diagnosis and management*. Chichester: John Wiley & Sons.

Edmonds ME, Foster AVM (2000). *Managing the Diabetic Foot*. Oxford: Blackwell Science.

Feher M (1993). *Hypertension in Diabetes Mellitus*. London: Martin Dunitz.

Foster MC, Cole M (1996). *Impotence: A guide to management*. London: Martin Dunitz.

Fox C, Pickering A (1995). *Diabetes in the Real World*. London: Class Publishing.

Gatling W, Hill R, Kirby M (1997) *Shared Care for Diabetes*. Oxford: ISIS Medical Media.

Hart JT, Fahey T, Savage W (1999). *High Blood Pressure at Your Fingertips*, 2nd edn. London: Class Publishing.

Hillson R (1996). *Diabetes: The complete guide*. London: Vermilion.

Jerreat L (1999). *Diabetes for Nurses*. London: Whurr Publishers.

MacKinnon M (2001). *Providing Diabetes Care in General Practice: A practical guide for the primary care team*, 4th edn. London: Class Publishing.

Pickup J, Williams G (1997). *Textbook of Diabetes*, 2nd edn. Oxford: Blackwell Science.

Shillitoe R (1994). *Counselling People with Diabetes*. Leicester: BPS Books.

Sönsken P, Fox C, Judd S (1998). *Diabetes at your Fingertips*, 4th edn. London: Class Publishing.

Watkins PJ, Drury PL, Howell SL (1996). *Diabetes and Its Management*, 5th edn. Oxford: Blackwell Science.

Williams G, Pickup J (1998). *Handbook of Diabetes*. Oxford: Blackwell Science.

Multimedia

Learning Diabetes (insulin treated) and *Learning Diabetes (non-insulin treated)*: multimedia patient education programmes produced as a package called Managing Your Health by Interactive Eurohealth. For information, please telephone, or fax, 01394 412141 or email sales@interactiveeurohealth.com

Journals

The Diabetic Foot
SB Communications Group*
Four issues per year.

Diabetic Medicine
Issued 12 times per year. Can be purchased through professional membership sections of Diabetes UK.

Diabetes and Primary Care
SB Communications Group*
Four issues per year.

Diabetes Update
Periodic newsletter (free) for healthcare professionals interested in diabetes; available for Diabetes UK members.

Journal of Diabetes Nursing
SB Communications Group*
Six issues per year.

Practical Diabetes International
Nine issues per year, available from John Wiley & Sons**.

* SB Communications Group, FREEPOST LON7814, London SE26 5BR.
** John Wiley & Sons, 1 Oldlands Way, Bognor Regis, W. Sussex PO22 9SA.

Companies and organisations

The following provide drugs, equipment, booklets, leaflets, posters, videos, identification cards, monitoring diaries, GP information training, clinic packs, etc. (local representatives will have specific details of what is available). Please contact them at the telephone numbers given to find out exactly what they do provide.

Diabetes UK

Diabetes UK is the national organisation for people with diabetes, with a section for primary care professionals, PCDUK. It is very useful first point of contact for all sorts of information and advice from welfare benefits to holidays. A publications list is available free from Diabetes UK:
0800 585088 (publications line).
10 Parkway,
London NW1 7AA
Tel: 020 7424 1000
Fax: 020 7424 1001
Email: info@diabetes.org.uk
Website: www.diabetes.org.uk
Some of the titles are free, but not all. The most widely used titles are:
Food Choices and Diabetes
Treating your Diabetes with
 Tablets
Coping with Diabetes When you
 are Ill
Diabetes: What care to expect

For specific cultural information, please ring the Health Care Delivery Department at Diabetes UK. Tel: 020 7323 1531; fax: 020 7637 3644

All primary care teams should join Diabetes UK (PCDUK).

3M Health Care Ltd
Tel: 01509 611611
Fax: 01509 237288

Aventis Pharma UK
Tel: 01732 584000
Fax: 01732 584080

Bayer plc
Tel: 01635 563000
Fax: 01635 566260
Helpline: 01635 566366

Becton Dickinson UK Ltd
Tel: 01865 781510
Fax: 01865 781551

Britannia Health Products
Tel: 01737 773741
Fax: 01737 773116

CP Pharmaceuticals
Tel: 01978 661261
Fax: 01978 660130

DVLA (Drivers and Vehicles Licensing Authority)
Medical Branch
Longview Road,
Swansea
SA99 1TU
Tel: 01792 772151
Fax: 01792 783779
Helpline: 0870 6000 301

Golden Key Company (SOS/Talisman)
Tel: 01795 663403
Fax: 01795 661356

GlaxoSmithKline
Tel: 020 8990 9000
Fax: 020 8990 4321

Hypoguard UK Ltd
Tel: 01394 387333/4
Fax: 01394 380152

LifeScan
Tel: 01494 450423
Fax: 01494 463299
Helpline: 0800 121200

Lilly Diabetes Care Division
Tel: 01256 315000
Fax: 01256 315058

Medic-Alert Foundation British Isles & Ireland
Tel: 020 7833 3034
Fax: 020 7278 0647
Helpline: 0800 581420

MediSense Britain Ltd
Tel: 01628 678900
Fax: 01628 678808
Helpline: 0500 467466

Merck Pharmaceuticals Ltd
Tel: 01895 452200
Fax: 01895 420605

Novo Nordisk Pharmaceuticals Ltd
Tel: 01293 613555
Fax: 01293 613535

Owen Mumford Ltd
Tel: 01993 812021
Fax: 01993 813466

Pfizer
Tel: 01304 616161
Fax: 01304 656221

Pharmacia Ltd
Tel: 01908 661101
Fax: 01908 690091

Quitline
(For help in stopping smoking)
Tel: 0800 002200

Roche Diagnostics
Tel: 01273 480444
Fax: 01273 480266
Direct Order Line: 0800 701000

Servier Laboratories Ltd
Tel: 01753 662744
Fax: 01753 663456

Smith & Nephew Health Care Ltd
Tel: 01482 222200
Fax: 01482 222211
Helpline: 0800 590173

Insurance and pensions

Diabetes UK Term Assurance Quoteline
Tel: 0800 731 7433

Diabetes UK Motor Quoteline
Tel: 0800 731 7432

Diabetes UK Travel Quoteline
Tel: 0800 731 7431

Devitt Insurance Services Ltd
Tel: 01708 385959
Fax: 0870 241 2358

Courses in academic institutions

English National Board Course No. 928 in Diabetic Nursing: details from the English National Board for Nursing, Midwifery and Health Visiting (see page 93).

Modules on diabetes: incorporated into other nursing courses: these are validated and may lead to a practice nurse attendance certificate/diploma or community nurse qualification/diploma.

Institutions offering courses:

- Colleges of nursing
- Colleges of health
- Institutes of health
- Colleges of further education
- Universities.

Distance learning courses

The mandatory training requirements for nurses for PREP (UKCC) are a total of 5 days over 3 years. For practice and continuity nurses, distance learning courses are popular. Apply to Diabetes UK for details of distance learning and other accredited courses.

Professional educational requirements

For nurses

- There are many developing diploma, degree and higher degree courses – in which diabetes may be a part or module.
- Credits or CAT points should be available on all validated courses where assessment is integral to the course.
- PREP and ENB Higher Award Schemes should make continuing education more available for all nurses.
- District diabetes care should include, in any strategy, the recognition of the need for local training and continuing education for nurses in primary care teams.
- Local or district schemes should be planned by specialist teams in conjunction with academic/continuing education institutions.

Short courses

Diabetic Course for Community Nurses
Department of Nursing and Midwifery, University of Glasgow, 68 Oakfield Avenue, Glasgow G12 8LS
Run twice a year. Contact Ms Joan McDowell, tel: 0141 339 8855

ENB 928 Short Course in Diabetic Nursing for Nurses, Midwives and Health Visitors on all Parts of the Professional Register
English National Board for Nursing, Midwifery and health Visiting, London
Courses run throughout the year; contact: NHS Careers, PO Box 376, Bristol BS99 3EY, tel: 0845 606 0655.

ENB AO5 The Care of Patients with Diabetes
60-day course run over a year.

ENB N97 Diabetes Nursing in Primary Health Care Settings
Course run over 25 days.

Multidisciplinary (certificate and diploma courses) (part distance learning)

Certificate in Diabetes Care
University of Warwick, Coventry CV4 7AL
Contact: Rachel Winnington, tel: 024 7657 2958

Diabetes Management in Primary Care (Diploma)
DTC Primary Care Training Centre, Shipley, W. Yorkshire
Run every 2 months; contact: Sarah Maylor, tel: 01274 617617

Working with Physical Illness: a systemic approach
Tavistock Clinic, London. Contact: Academic Services, tel: 020 7447 3718

Working with Families and Teams – an introduction to systems-based approaches in general practice
Tavistock Clinic, London. Contact: Academic Services, tel: 020 7447 3718

Masters courses over a longer period

Postgraduate Diploma in Diabetes Care for Healthcare Professionals
University of Exeter
Module programme of two taught and one self-directed learning modules (one day per week). Run over one year; contact: Mrs Peta Fenn, Institute of General Practice, University of Exeter

Masters in Clinical Science (Diabetes)
University of Warwick, Coventry, CV4 7AL
Modular diabetes diploma and masters courses (with modules as stand-alone postgraduate awards) for health care professionals. These courses will become available in October 2001. For information contact: Warwick Diabetes Care, tel: 024 7657 2958

Graduate Certificated/Graduate Diploma/Masters in Diabetes
Chelsea & Westminster Hospital, 369 Fulham Road, London/University of Surrey, Roehampton. Run once a year, also run a distance learning course; contact: Helen Laird, tel: 020 8237 2731 or Patricia O'Connell, tel: 020 8392 3562.

Feedback Form

We, the authors, would welcome your comments on this second edition.
Would you like more on some subjects and less on others?
Are there additional topics which you would like to see in future editions?
Please help us by marking your comments on this page, cutting it out
or photocopying it, and sending it to the publisher, postfree, at
Class Publishing, FREEPOST, London W6 7BR

Current topics   **More?**   **Less?**

1: *Impact and new insights*   ☐   ☐
2: *Screening and identification*   ☐   ☐
3: *How to manage type 2 diabetes*   ☐   ☐
4: *How to control blood glucose levels*   ☐   ☐
5: *How to reduce long-term complications of diabetes*   ☐   ☐
6: *How to manage type 1 diabetes*   ☐   ☐
7: *How to manage pregnancy and gestational diabetes*   ☐   ☐
8: *Living with diabetes*   ☐   ☐
9: *Emergencies and illness*   ☐   ☐
10: *Monitoring care in the practice*   ☐   ☐

Additional topics

....

....

....

Other comments

....

....

....

May we contact you?

Name: *Occupation:*

Address:

....

Town: *Postcode:*

Priority Order Form

Please cut out or photocopy this form and send it to:
Class Publishing (Priority Service)
FREEPOST (*no stamp required if posted in the UK*), **London W6 7BR**

***URGENT** – please send me the following books: (tick boxes below)*

No. of copies		*Price including p&p*
____ *Vital diabetes* (1 872362 93 1)		£17.99
____ *Diabetes in the real world* (1 872362 53 2)		£22.95
____ *Providing diabetes care in general practice* (1 85959 048 9)		£24.95
____ *Diabetes at your fingertips* (1 872362 79 6)		£17.99
____ *High blood pressure at your fingertips* (1 872362 81 8)		£17.99

____ Please send me the new 3rd edition of *Vital Diabetes*, with an invoice, when it is published in 2002.

____ Please send me further details about these books

Please note all prices include UK postage and handling costs.

For express service, use our Hotlines:

Tel: 01752 202 301   Fax: 01752 202 333

EASY WAYS TO PAY

1. I enclose a cheque made payable to Class Publishing for _____

2. Please charge my   Access ☐   Visa ☐   Switch ☐   Amex ☐

Card No. _____ *Expiry date* _____

Name _____ *Occupation* _____

Delivery address _____

_____

Daytime telephone (in case of query) _____

Send to: **Class Publishing (Priority Service), FREEPOST, London W6 7BR**
Or use one of the Hotlines listed above

Publisher's no quibble guarantee: your money back if you are not entirely satisfied, within 30 days.